EVEN IF YOU EAT A BALANCED DIET, YOU MAY NOT BE MEETING YOUR NUTRITIONAL NEEDS!

- Spinach can lose half of its vitamin C when stored at room temperature for three days
- Lettuce can lose a fourth of its vitamins A and C in a few days even when refrigerated properly
- Instant potatoes have virtually no vitamin C at all, unlike fresh potatoes, which contain appreciable vitamin C
- Freshly squeezed orange juice can lose 2% of its vitamin C each day in your refrigerator
- Fresh-cooked foods can lose up to 56% of their nutrients in cooking
- Canned foods lose 30% of their nutrients in the scalding process, 25% in sterilization, 27% in liquor diffusion, and 12% in reheating
- Frozen foods lose 25% of their nutrients in the scalding process, 19% in freezing, 15% in thawing and 24% in cooking

Let Richard A. Passwater, Ph.D., Director of the Solgar Nutritional Research Center, show you how to make sure you get all the nutrients you need for optimal health with . . .

THE NEW SUPERNUTRITION

THE NEW SUPER-NUTRITION

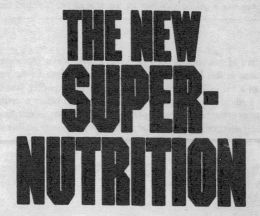

RICHARD A. PASSWATER, Ph.D.

POCKET BOOKS

New York   London   Toronto   Sydney   Tokyo   Singapore

The author of this book is not a physician and the ideas, procedures and suggestions in this book are not intended as a substitute for the medical advice of a trained health professional. All matters regarding your health require medical supervision. Consult your physician before adopting the suggestions in this book, as well as any condition that may require diagnosis or medical attention. The author and publishers disclaim any liability arising directly or indirectly from the use of this book.

An *Original* Publication of POCKET BOOKS

POCKET BOOKS, a division of Simon & Schuster Inc.
1230 Avenue of the Americas, New York, NY 10020

Copyright © 1991 by Richard A. Passwater

ISBN: 0-671-70071-5

First Pocket Books printing May 1991

10 9 8 7 6 5 4

POCKET and colophon are registered trademarks of Simon & Schuster Inc.

Printed in the U.S.A.

Contents

■

III SUPERNUTRITION AGAINST CANCER

■

IV SUPERNUTRITION AGAINST HEART DISEASE

■

V SUPERNUTRITION AGAINST OTHER NON-GERM DISEASES

VI COMPLETING THE SUPERNUTRITION STORY

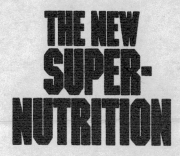

THE NEW SUPER-NUTRITION

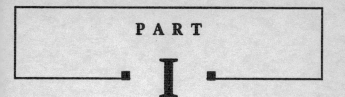

PART

I

The Foundations
of
Supernutrition

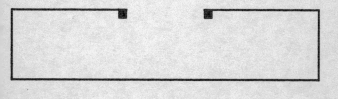

1

Supernutrition

The U.S. government has finally made disease prevention its main health goal! On September 6, 1990, Secretary of Health and Human Services Louis Sullivan announced the U.S. government's prescription for a healthier nation by the year 2000—"take responsibility for your own health and life-style." The United States' number-one health official added, "We can no longer afford to ignore the fact that prevention is the single most important factor in maintaining good health. Control of key risk factors could prevent up to 70% of premature deaths."

That's what this book is all about—preventing disease, improving health and the quality of life. It has taken the government a long time to realize it, but disease prevention can be achieved easily with better nutrition and improved life-style. This has been the focus of my laboratory research and writing for over twenty-five years. As Dr. J. Michael McGinnis of the Office of Disease Prevention and Health Promotion said, "The focus on prevention represents a major change in the government's attitude toward disease."

The New Supernutrition shows you how best to prevent

disease and improve your health with easy steps that are tailored to the way *you* do things. You know what you are willing to change, and you know what you are never going to give up. Here are some new steps that you can add to improve your health, even when you can't bring yourself to do all those things that you "know you should."

The New Supernutrition customizes your diet and supplement program to produce the best possible health for *you*. *The New Supernutrition* is your guide to maximum energy. *The New Supernutrition* doesn't rely on averages for large populations of persons genetically different from you. *The New Supernutrition* considers all health issues including the avoidance of cancer and heart disease and the slowing of the aging process. *The New Supernutrition* is not merely concerned with average health but utilizes modern nutritional science and my research to supercharge you to all that you can be and want to be.

During the late 1960s four researchers independently arrived at new nutritional principles that brought improved health to many. Dr. Linus Pauling developed the concept of "orthomolecular medicine." This loosely means "the right molecule in the right concentrations at the right time for the best health."[1]

Dr. Roger Williams completed his concept of "biochemical individuality." Biochemical individuality recognizes that each of us is extraordinary and has specific nutrient needs due to genetic factors that differ from the average.[2]

Dr. Emanuel Cheraskin developed the concept of "optimal dietary intake." This concept recognizes the truism that there is a nutrient intake level that produces above-average health.[3] And lastly, and I hope not least, I developed the concept of "Supernutrition." Supernutrition, in essence, is similar to Dr. Cheraskin's Optimal Dietary Intake.[4] Dr. Cheraskin's approach was retrospective, while mine was prospective.

Although the four of us became friends, our work at that time was independent. Later we would share and compare notes as each reinforced the work of the others. We were all approaching the same goal from different directions. I was a gerontologist conducting laboratory animal experiments to slow the aging process and prevent cancer.

Dr. Pauling became interested in man's missing enzyme system that prevents us from making our own vitamin C like most other animals do. He was very curious as to how the genetic defect and dependence on dietary vitamin C affected human health.

Dr. Williams had long ago noticed the physical differences in body organs. He wondered if the physical differences were also accompanied by biochemical differences. In medical school he noticed in surgery that the classic organs shown in textbook illustrations were seldom found. Instead of the stomach we see in TV antacid commercials he found a dozen distinct types, each having many variations. Similarly, when Dr. Williams measured biochemical levels of many enzymes in the body he found great variations.

Now there are many researchers looking into the relationships of genetics and biochemical variation.[5] Not only are differences in nutrient requirements being studied, but so are differences in food preferences.

Dr. Luigi Cavalli-Sforza of Stanford has found that genetic transmission of food preferences tends to remain very stable over time. Dr. Adam Drewnowski of the University of Michigan discovered that genetic influence on taste perception may be far-reaching and may ultimately be linked to chronic disease risk.

Others found there were genetic determinants for food sensitivities, tolerances, and allergies, which confirms Dr. Williams's findings. Dr. Daniel Rudman of the Medical College of Wisconsin declared that nutrient thresholds—the minimal requirement or maximal tolerance for essential nutrients—are also influenced by genetic programming. The ability to absorb and conserve nutrients has a genetic base and also affects nutrient thresholds.

In some cases thresholds are drastically altered by inherited metabolic characteristics, such as inborn errors of amino acid and carbohydrate metabolism, salt-sensitive hypertension, familial hyperlipidemias, and type II diabetes mellitus. The aging process, which Dr. Rudman says is "nutritionally determined," can also alter nutrient thresholds.

Dr. Howard Schneider of the University of North Carolina states, "A new paradigm is needed. One feature of the new paradigm will be a recognition of genetic variability in the population, and of the interactions of genotype and environment (including especially the nutritional environment) which affect the human condition."[6]

Dr. Cheraskin sought reasons explaining the various levels of health that exist. He noticed that it was not a matter of people being either healthy or sick. Some were very healthy and superenergetic; others were of average health; some were always a little "sub-par"; and a percentage were always sickly. Dr. Cheraskin examined their diets and found that the healthiest were usually those eating the foods with the highest levels of vitamins and minerals.

All research paths confirmed the principle of supernutrition: that an optimal nutrient intake exists for many of us different from the standard recommended dietary intakes. Supernutrition is designed to determine *your* best vitamin and mineral intake.

I'll document what I say in this book so you can read more about research of particular interest, and so skeptics can check the facts. I used this tactic successfully to get other scientists interested in slowing the aging process and preventing cancer. When I lecture I challenge the audience to prove me wrong by conducting their own research. Then I explain my research and encourage them to investigate on their own. At first there were those so eager to prove me wrong that they rushed to their labs and replicated my experiments. When they verified my results they soon became engrossed in newer and better experiments extending my findings.

For example, Dr. Cheraskin determined Optimal Dietary Intakes by comparing dietary intakes with levels of health. This is retrospective and often used by epidemiologists to see if a concept warrants further study. He looked at the clinical history of people and then analyzed their diets. He found that those with the fewest clinical symptoms had the highest intake of vitamins and minerals. The intakes of vitamins and minerals that produced the best health were nearly the same as the Supernutrition levels.

I determined the Supernutrition values first by laboratory animal experiments and then by trial and response with volunteers. This is prospective rather than retrospective and considered the most accurate method by which to verify a concept.

In the twenty-first century we will see more health advances as people realize the value of trace minerals and food factors that most haven't even heard of yet. You can start your New Supernutrition Plan in the 1990s.

2

Goals

The New Supernutrition brings about improved health by better nourishment of each cell in the body. This is not a medical book. The emphasis is on preventing health problems, but many people respond so quickly to improved nutrition that they call the change miraculous. Although I received many hundreds of letters claiming miraculous improvements in health from readers of *Supernutrition,* this book is not intended to miraculously cure disease.

The point of *The New Supernutrition,* as in *Supernutrition,* is to find the best vitamin and mineral intake to produce the best health. This is not an endorsement of just taking large amounts of supplements. It is an endorsement of taking the right amount, whatever that amount turns out to be.

A later section of the book guides you in determining your optimal nutrient intake. This is the New Supernutrition Plan. Some people who never read *Supernutrition* just assumed that I recommended the highest level of vitamins and minerals that was safe to take. Not so! There is no need to take more than the amount that lets your body be as healthy as it can be.

If the goal were merely to recommend high levels of supplements, a simple chart listing those quantities would do. Chapter 41 gives you guidelines according to your age, diet, and life-style, plus each chapter gives a summary of nutrient intake that applies to a "typical" health problem. As an example, if you wish to lower your cholesterol level, a range of nutrient levels is given that studies show to be effective for most people. Your best range of nutrient intake is suggested by the higher range of the two, not by adding the two together.

Besides helping you determine your best nutrient intake, I will bring you up to date on the latest research on diet and disease relationships. In addition to my own research at the Solgar Nutritional Research Center on slowing aging and preventing cancer and heart disease, I will discuss the most promising research of others. It is difficult to measure your progress in preventing disease, so you should know what research shows to be preventative. You should realize there are alternate ways to achieve the goal of optimal health. You may find that one program better suits your life-style than another, yet the result will be the same.

Rather than just giving you recommendations, I will discuss the research so you can better understand how each alternative approach works.

In addition, there is a handy reference section giving facts about the purpose, use, and safety of each nutrient. Several of the nutrients in the New Supernutrition may be new to you. You will find additional information about these nutrients in various chapters. You may want to keep this book on hand as a reference even long after you have determined your optimal supplement program.

The concepts presented here will be new to many in the field of dietetics and medicine. Some members of these professions have historically labeled anything new or not understood by them as faddism or quackery. Many of these critics are the same ones who have planned the horrible hospital menus that lead to malnutrition for 50,000 hospitalized patients each year,[1-6] in spite of studies published for more than twenty years in medical journals complaining about hospital-dietician-induced malnutrition.[7]

Please do not confuse nutritional advice with medical treatment. The emphasis of this book is on health and prevention, not the diagnosis, treatment, and cure of existing disease. This is the realm of physicians. This is not to say that the information given in this book will not help cure any health problem. Better nutrition is a perfect adjunct to any medical treatment. It is easier to cure a person with a healthy immune system and organ system reserve than to try to cure a poorly nourished, sickly body. It makes all the difference in the world.

One principle that I always insist upon: Do not delay getting your physician's evaluation if you feel ill or have clinical symptoms. Do *not* try to see if a better diet will take care of the problem. If it doesn't, you may have lost valuable time, and it may be too late. First get a medical evaluation. Then add better nourishment as an adjunct.

You are responsible for your own health. Take advantage of the best of what each health care professional can provide you. Utilize good medical advice and good nutritional advice. They are complementary—not competitive.

3

The Need for Supernutrition

Even those in "perfect health" can benefit from *The New Supernutrition*. They can correct unrecognized deficiencies of the newly discovered nutrients before irreversible symptoms develop.

In 1975 *Supernutrition* explained how antioxidant nutrients destroy free radicals that speed aging and cause diseases including cancer and heart disease. This was new information to nutritionists and physicians as well as to the public. Now the role of antioxidant nutrients in free-radical pathology is well proven and accepted.

Supernutrition introduced new nutrients such as selenium and dimethylglycine.

In 1977 *Supernutrition for Healthy Hearts* introduced high-density lipoprotein (HDL) cholesterol—the "good cholesterol"—and low-density lipoprotein (LDL)—the "bad cholesterol." Also, the role of free radicals in causing heart disease by monoclonal proliferation was discussed.

In 1988 the New York Academy of Sciences held a seminar that presented scores of studies showing that vitamin E was effective in preventing or treating chronic disease, including heart disease and cancer.

Also in 1988 the Centers for Disease Control reported that women who took multivitamin supplements around the time of conception had babies with fewer birth defects. The *Journal of the American Medical Association* published an editorial for women to "hear and follow this simple advice."

I will update my research in this book. There are several new concepts and alternative health strategies that you should know about. Now that we understand more about preventing heart disease, it is clear that blood cholesterol levels are only a part of the story. The role of trace minerals and new vitaminlike factors are more important.

The newer nutrients have vital roles in slowing aging, preventing cancer, and improving overall health and energy. These trace nutrients can correct previously unexplained maladies and energy loss. They improve health to a new level.

The typical American is not even nourished to the "adequate" level that the RDA committee strives for, let alone the optimal level. That's hard to believe, especially when there are so many rewards for good health.

Undernourished Americans

A recent study by the National Cancer Institute found that 40% of Americans don't eat a single fruit and 20% don't have a vegetable on a typical day.[1] Fifty-one percent don't eat a vegetable other than potatoes and salads. Eighty percent eat no high-fiber cereal or whole-grain breads.

One in four of us skips breakfast. The Council for Responsible Nutrition notes, "the USDA National Food Consumption Survey showed that only 3% of the population ate diets which met the Four Food Groups pattern, and only 12% obtained 100% of the RDA for each of SEVEN nutrients. NOT A SINGLE PERSON of the more than 21,500 people surveyed OBTAINED 100% OF THE RDA FOR EACH OF TEN NUTRIENTS.[2] This trend has been developing for decades. In 1952 the U.S. Public Health Service survey disclosed that more than one thousand of our daily calories came from foods devoid of protein, vitamins, and minerals.[3] These are the so-called "empty calorie" foods.

A U.S. Department of Agriculture study in 1977 and 1978 of eleven of the twenty-eight micronutrients found that at least one third of us consumed less than 70% of the government's recommendation for calcium, iron, magnesium, and vitamin B-6.[4] This occurred throughout all socioeconomic groups.

Girls fifteen to seventeen years of age on low-calorie diets met the RDA for only one nutrient. Only one person in five obtained the RDA of vitamin B-6, and one person out of two ate less than 70% of the RDA of vitamin B-6. Calcium was a problem nutrient for half of American women.

One third of all persons studied had vitamin A intakes below 70% of the RDA. One fourth had vitamin C intakes below 70% of the RDA. More than 40% had calcium intakes less than 70% of the RDA.

Thirty-one percent got less than 70% of the RDA for vitamin A. The National Academy of Sciences, the National Cancer Institute, and the American Cancer Society believe vitamin A helps prevent cancer.

A USDA researcher pointed out in 1985 that nine out of ten Americans do not get enough of the mineral chromium.[5] Another 1985 USDA study found that vitamin and mineral intakes had not changed much since their 1977–78 study.[6] Vitamin B-6 and folic acid intakes had dropped for women, who averaged only 61% of the vitamin B-6 RDA and 51% of the folic acid RDA.

In 1985 women were averaging 60% of the zinc RDA, 61% of the iron RDA, and 78% of the calcium RDA. A similar study by the FDA found that Americans were eating low levels of calcium, magnesium, zinc, iron, copper, and manganese. Of course, neither of these two studies considered selenium, chromium, or other important trace minerals.

Many experts feel that the recommended amounts are too low. People may be living longer on the average, but many are in poor health. If more people could get the optimum levels of vitamins and minerals, then people would have a longer prime of life and better health longer.

Table 3.1 list the results of surveys for four vitamins and two minerals taken through the years. Table 3.2 shows the percentage of people getting less than the RDA for the "easy to get" vitamins and minerals in 1980.

TABLE 3.1
The results of surveys through the years illustrate how poorly Americans nourish themselves

Nutrient	% not getting the RDA*			
	1955	1965	1970	1980
Vitamin A	20	26	50	55
Vitamin B-1	5	8	45	50
Vitamin B-2	5	6	34	38
Vitamin C	22	27	41	52
Calcium	20	30	68	73
Iron	10	10	57	59

*RDA levels change through the years

TABLE 3.2
Percentage of people getting less than the RDA for the "easy-to-get" vitamins and nutrients

Nutrient	% not getting RDA
Vitamin B-6	80
Magnesium	75
Calcium	68
Iron	57
Vitamin A	50
Vitamin B-1	45
Vitamin C	41
Vitamin B-2	34
Vitamin B-12	34
Vitamin B-3	33

USDA study of 40,000 Americans—Nationwide Food Consumption Survey. See *Food Technology* 35:9, 1981.

Wrong Choices

People have not been getting the recommended amounts of many nutrients. The Council for Responsible Nutrition finds that 97% of Americans do not eat diets that match the RDA.

As people become less active they reduce their food intake in an attempt to maintain desired body weight. The best way of putting the necessary nutrients into a reduced-calorie diet is with vitamin and mineral supplements.

Why would educated people or people who could afford to eat almost anything they want shorten their lives by eating so poorly?

Actually, the educated affluent have heard only part of the nutrition story. They are trying to live longer by cutting fats and cholesterol from their diets. Attempts to avoid certain foods bring about nutritional problems because these are often the foods that are rich in trace nutrients. Foodstuffs that are egg substitutes, butter substitutes, cheese substitutes, milk substitutes, and meat substitutes are not rich in vitamins and minerals.

The educated affluent are also busy people. Convenience foods are usually overprocessed or overcooked and are frequently "empty calorie" foods. People know they can't rely too much on convenience foods, but their life-style allows little choice too much of the time.

Conventional Advice Is Not Good Enough

It's good advice to eat a varied diet in moderation from among the four food groups. Don't eat too much of any one food, and don't be afraid to eat any whole food unless you are allergic to it. Don't eat more calories than required to maintain ideal body weight.

As good as that advice sounds, it isn't good enough. It does not ensure a "balanced diet" or optimal nutrition.

A study conducted at Pennsylvania State University found that the recommended portions of the "basic four" food groups do not ensure adequate amounts of essential nutrients.[7] Particular problems were found with vitamin E, vitamin B-6, iron, zinc, magnesium, and folic acid. The study did not include trace minerals such as selenium and chromium.

In the study, forty-six adult volunteers meticulously selected the recommended number of servings from the four basic food groups. In spite of their diligence in following the

TABLE 3.3
The "Balanced" Diet

Group	Servings	Percentage
Cereals/grains	4	34
Fruits/vegetables	4	34
Dairy	2	16
Meats/legumes	2	16

Nutritionists use a simplified approach to teach a "balanced" diet. Specific serving sizes from four basic food groups help teach some perspective, especially if variety is used within those groups. However, even this approach does not ensure a diet that meets the Recommended Dietary Allowances.

TABLE 3.4
The "SAD" Diet

Group	Percentage
Cereals/grain	7.6
Fruits/vegetables	20.8
Dairy	18.8
Meats/legumes	16.0
Others	38.8

The Standard American Diet (SAD) still doesn't meet the ideal diet, even after decades of teaching the "basic four" groups. It's hard to get people to eat what they don't "want," even if they know it's better for them. The solution is to work within this truism and add better nourishment to what people are really eating while trying to teach the benefits of improving food selection. Food supplements help achieve this goal. The best answer is better food selection along with supplements to replace lost nutrients.

rules, 67% did not receive the recommended amounts of vitamins E and B-6, iron, and zinc. A third also came up short of the RDA for magnesium and folic acid.

This problem was addressed by French nutritionist Dr. Jean-Pierre Mareschi. "The 'balanced diet' is a diet based on the selection of a wide range of food products and on the knowledge of the various body requirements, and which aims at meeting these requirements. 'At risk' nutrients are those present in the balanced diet in amounts below 80% of

TABLE 3.5
United States Dietary Trends 1860–1975

	% of energy from major nutrients			
	1860	1920	1925	1975
Protein	12	12	12	12–15
Fat	25	32	35	40–45
Carbohydrates				
Complex (starches)	53	43	37	22
Simple (sugars)	10	13	16	24
Total carbohydrate	63	56	53	46

The trends of the "macro" nutrients (after Burkett, H. C., and Trowell, H. C., in *Western Diseases: Their Emergence and Prevention* (Cambridge, MA: Harvard University Press, 1981).

the recommended levels, when calorie intake is normal. *If a population is found to be low in 'at risk' nutrients, eating a balanced diet cannot be relied on to correct the problem.*"[8]

In the French population Dr. Mareschi identifies vitamins B-1, B-2, B-5, B-6, and E, and folic acid, plus the minerals iron, copper, zinc, iodine, and manganese. Remember, this applies to a *balanced* diet. The condition is much worse for "typical" diets.

Another problem with the basic four food groups is that several new foodstuffs are difficult to place into the system. Also, few people can remember the proper portions from each group needed to balance the diet.

Table 3.3 shows what the percentages of macronutrients should be according to many nutritionists. Table 3.4 shows the actual average diet. No wonder there are so many deficiencies of the vitamin and mineral micronutrients, when the macronutrients aren't even close to balance. Table 3.5 shows diet composition through many decades.

We can't blame it all on poor nutritional education! Many prefer "empty calorie" and high-fat foods.

Disappearing Nutrients

Even when we select the proper foods, the nutrients we expect to be there are not there. Food tables list certain levels of vitamins and minerals for foods, but foods differ from the "book values." Variety differences, depleted soils, harvesting before maturation, loss during transportation, storage losses, processing losses, cooking losses, and waste account for the difference.

Another difference from book value is due to bio-availability. Bioavailability determines the amount of a nutrient in a food that gets into your body. As an example, the calcium listed for spinach is largely an insoluble oxalate salt. The body poorly absorbs insoluble mineral salts. Foods differ widely in the bioavailability of their vitamins and minerals.

Consumer taste preferences dictate which varieties of fruits and vegetables are grown, and better-tasting varieties are always being developed. However, the book values for nutrients in these foods don't keep pace with the changing varieties. As an example, Silver Queen white sweet corn doesn't have the same vitamin A content as the older, more yellow, less sugary variety listed in the food table. French beans can vary as much as 2,000% in vitamin B-2 levels. Whole wheat germ can vary by 500% in vitamin B-1 levels.

Commercial fertilizers do not replace all the minerals depleted from overused soils. Also, changes in soil mineral balance affect which minerals are taken up by the plants. Soils with sulfur deficiencies reduce the amount of iron and manganese absorbed by the plants. Soil that has too much sulfur due to acid rain reduces the amount of selenium absorbed by the plant. As an example, the selenium content of wheat can vary by a factor of one thousand in crops grown less than a mile apart.

Poor storage during transportation also reduces the vitamin content of foods. You can't be sure if the food you buy was properly refrigerated at all times during transportation. Some foods such as apples and potatoes are stored for more than six months before being used. Do you know how to select the freshest fruits and vegetables? Unless you grow your own, you can't be sure of freshness.

Spinach can lose half of its vitamin C when stored at room temperature for three days.[9] Lettuce can lose a fourth of its vitamin A and vitamin C in a few days even when refrigerated properly.[10]

Another type of storage and processing destroys much of the vitamin content of reconstituted foods. Potatoes reconstituted from instant mixes have virtually no vitamin C at all, yet fresh potatoes are a decent source of vitamin C.

Orange juice stored in cardboard cartons has only 70% of the vitamin C in fresh-squeezed orange juice, and orange juice stored in glass bottles has only 60% of the vitamin C of fresh juice. Freshly squeezed orange juice can lose 2% of its vitamin C each day it is in your refrigerator.[11]

Even frozen foods continue to lose vitamins. At 0°F more than 50% of the vitamin C is lost from some frozen vegetables in slightly more than six months.[12] Even at −5° the same vegetables lose 20% of their vitamin C in the same period of time.

Forty percent of the vitamin A, 100% of the vitamin C, 80% of the B-complex, and 55% of the vitamin E can be lost during the processing, storage, and heating of TV dinners.

The processing of foods—such as milling, canning, freezing, and cooking—destroys vitamins and minerals. An analysis of 723 foods showed that canning can destroy as much as 77% of the vitamin B-6, 78% of the vitamin B-5, and much of the biotin and folic acid. Even minerals are lost in the canning process. Canned spinach, canned beans, and canned tomatoes lose 40%, 60%, and 83% of the zinc that was present when they were fresh.[13]

Peas cooked garden-fresh lose 56% of their vitamins by serving time; but canned peas lose 94%, and frozen peas lose 83%.

Table 3.6 shows some of the nutrient losses in foods.

You can never be sure just what the vitamin and mineral content of a food is. Book values are a guide, but actual food servings can vary by a factor of a thousand from the book value.

One way to be sure that you are getting an adequate nutrient intake is to take vitamin and mineral supplements

TABLE 3.6
Nutrient Losses from Foods

Cooked Fresh	56% in cooking
Canned	30% in the scalding process
	25% in the sterilization process
	27% in the liquor diffusion
	12% in reheating
Frozen	25% in the scalding process
	19% in the freezing process
	15% in the thawing process
	24% in cooking

along with your meals—even if the meals consist of the proper portions of the four basic food groups.

Table 3.7 shows the amounts of several vitamins lost in the canning process.[14]

All grains are processed to some degree before we eat them. Each stage of the process destroys nutrients. Whole grains have more nutrients than white flours. Grains have four layers: husk, bran, endosperm, and germ. The germ has the most nutrients but spoils easily. Thus, processors like to remove the germ so that the flour can be stored longer.

Milling takes at least twenty nutrients out of wheat. White bread has only 20% of the zinc, 25% of the iron, 30% of the chromium, 40% of the calcium, and 60% of the magnesium of whole wheat bread.[15] Milling removes 86% of the vitamin E, 80% of the vitamin B-3, 75% of the vitamin B-6, 67% of the folic acid, and 50% of the vitamin B-5 of whole wheat bread.

Enrichment doesn't make up for the loss due to food processing. Processors may point out that the milled flour is "enriched," but this only means that four vitamins and two minerals are added back. Even then they are not returned to their original levels.

Cooking destroys vitamins and minerals. The cutting of food alone starts enzymatic reactions and oxidation that destroy vitamins. Overcooking or reheating destroys more than 80% of certain vitamins.[16]

TABLE 3.7
Canning Destroys Vitamins

Vitamin	% Destroyed
Vitamin A	39
Vitamin B-1	69
Vitamin B-2	55
Vitamin B-3	46
Vitamin B-6	54
Folic acid	61
Pantothenic acid	61
Biotin	51
Vitamin C	64

The several stages of the canning process destroy a significant portion of many vitamins. Unless you eat more than the ideal portions to maintain your desired weight, then you may wish to consider replacing the lost vitamins with vitamin supplements.

The average loss of minerals from vegetables is calcium, 32%; magnesium, 45%; phosphorus, 46%; and iron, 48%.[17] Much of the vitamin and mineral content of a food can be drained away and thrown out with the cooking water or peeled and thrown away in the skin.

Heating destroys the vitamin C in tomato juice. Cooking or processing tomato juice at 220°F destroys 60% of its original vitamin C.

Adding baking soda to peas to intensify their color destroys much of the vitamin B-1 and vitamin C. Sulfites make salads look better longer, but they also destroy vitamins.

You never can really tell if you are getting everything the books say are in various foods.

To get foods to the market before they rot, growers harvest them prematurely and artificially "ripen" them at the right time so they will look fresh at the market. This ripening process gives appropriate color and flavor but doesn't give the vitamin content that natural "vine" ripening develops.

Persons in apparently good health will benefit from nutrient optimization. If they are slightly deficient in any nutrient—even in one of the newer ones that they haven't heard of yet—they will begin the cascade downward to poorer health. Let's examine how nutrient deficiencies relate to the various stages of health and sickness.

There are several reasons for stressing nutritional supplements rather than foods rich in the critical nutrients. Of course, wherever possible you should try to get the nutrients in a varied, balanced diet or add certain nutrient-rich foods to your diet. Just about everyone has heard this message, but a Gallup Poll sponsored by the American Dietetic Association and the International Food Information Council found that just 8% of us are eating more vegetables and only 6% are consuming more fruits and fruit juices. Here are some of the reasons for stressing the supplements:

(1) It's impossible to know how much of the newly discovered nutrients are in the foods because food tables have not yet been prepared that include these new nutrients.

(2) In order to get adequate amounts of some of the trace nutrients, the natural food sources must be concentrated. An alternative would be to eat lots of those foods, but the calories would be excessive.

(3) Several rich sources of the critical nutrients are food forms not in conventional diets. Also, people tend to tire of such foods rapidly. As an example, a nutrient found in fatty fish protects against heart disease. Can you eat mackerel four times a week? Would you rather take a tasteless capsule?

(4) You may have already chosen not to change your diet, but you might consider adding supplements.

(5) You are too busy to prepare new foods, and you want the convenience of supplements. The ultimate convenience for busy people is food supplements in pill form. They are premeasured, inexpensive, tasteless, and compatible with your favorite meals.

The last two reasons may not seem valid to those who practice what they believe to be perfect nutritional habits, but many of us in the real world have already decided that we are set in our eating habits. We need whatever help we can get. So what if our nutritional shortcuts end up giving us better health than that obtained by those who follow the prudent—but alas, imperfect—diet?

4

Superhealth

Your nutrient level determines how healthy you are. Undernutrition impairs your immune system. Undernutrition saps your energy. Trace-nutrient deficiencies can make you fat.

The converse is also true. Optimal nourishment will supercharge you, help protect you from disease, and normalize your appetite. Superhealth is the world's greatest aphrodisiac.

Although these newly discovered nutrients are of paramount importance for protection from major diseases, it could be ten years before health professionals apply them to the treatment of patients.

The knowledge gained in the 1970s involving the protective role of trace minerals against cancer and heart disease is just beginning to be applied in daily medical practice. However, trace minerals are not taken into account by those still thinking about "balanced" diets only in terms of fats, carbohydrates and proteins.

The main problem of trace-nutrient deficiency is that it can eventually destroy your health. Without good health you have nothing.

The small gap between what you need and what you get adds up just like your bank account. If you don't make as much money as you need, eventually you will become bankrupt. It doesn't matter if it occurs with a big deficit in a short time or a small deficit over a long period. If you run out of reserves, you become bankrupt. The main problem with trace-nutrient deficiency is that it will eventually cause health bankruptcy.

The deficiency can become more serious than just fatigue or weight gain. You can't always tell that the nutritional deficiency is changing from a chronic condition to an acute condition. Then it may be too late to reverse its progress. A healthy immune system can destroy an isolated cancer cell or two. However, if a cancer-causing agent mutates a cell while your immune system is weak, it may develop into a noncurable cancer.

The same is true for many other diseases in addition to the classical deficiency diseases.

Nutritional deficiencies go through five recognized stages in the chain of events leading to disease. Your body does not exist in one of two stages—either being healthy or ill. There are many stages of good health and illness.

There are five recognized depletion stages: hidden hunger, marginal deficiency, subclinical, clinical, and terminal. These stages are also called preliminary, biochemical, physiological, clinical, and terminal.

The first event in the sequence that leads to poor health is a preliminary stage where the nutritional gap causes the body to use up any stores of nutrients it may have. This first stage also slows the elimination of nutrients from the body. It is a good sign when you are excreting nutrients because that is assurance that you are not depleting your emergency store of nutrients.

The second event in the sequence leading to illness is the biochemical stage. In this stage there is a reduced level of action by the compounds that regulate thousands of biochemical reactions in the body. Compounds called "enzymes" regulate most of our body's chemistry. Thousands of these enzymes have a member of the vitamin B family incorporated into their structure.

If you become vitamin B deficient, you don't make as many of the needed enzymes. The resulting deficiency in enzymes first slows body chemistry, then alters it. In this second stage of deficiency the excretion of nutrients reaches its minimal level.

The third stage of deficiency is called the physiological level or subclinical stage. In the third stage behavioral effects such as irritability, personality changes, reduced resistance to disease, and weight changes occur. Also, the changes observed in stage two occur with greater severity. This stage sends people to physicians with multiple and vague symptoms. However, few doctors are trained to recognize or distinguish these symptoms from those of other diseases.

The fourth stage of nutritional deficiency is the clinical stage in which the classic symptoms of nutritional diseases appear. What earlier was the tiredness and irritability of a marginal deficiency of vitamin B-1 or B-3 is now beriberi or pellagra.

The final stage is the terminal stage, in which there is severe tissue damage resulting in death unless corrected. Fortunately, stages four and five are fairly rare in the United States, Canada, and Europe.

By not getting the recommended amounts of vitamins and nutrients, you can be less healthy than you want to be.

Small deficiencies can bring on severe illness. Malnourishment can lead to death in other ways than classical malnutrition. Marginal deficiencies lead to an impaired immune response, which means increased susceptibility to disease and infection. It also means that marginal deficiencies impair the power of the body to recover from disease or infection. There is growing evidence that nutrients are involved in our resistance to cancer and heart disease.

The average person can't see this relationship because it's hard to tie the effect and cause together. The disease doesn't show up right after a poor meal.

Most people understand how important the right gasoline is to their car and the value of good materials in construction. That is because we can readily see the results. Nutrition is much more complex. Changes show up after years of abuse, not immediately after a meal.

Vitamins are more than spark plugs unleashing energy from food the way a real spark plug releases the energy in gasoline. A spark plug may deliver just a little spark, but the energy released by the explosion of the gasoline is powerful.

If the spark is missing, the engine "misses" and runs with poor efficiency and little power.

Vitamins have many roles in the body. We are discovering more roles as science moves on. Some vitamins carry out specific body chemical reactions such as releasing the energy in food or breaking down fat molecules. Other vitamins protect cells against the damage that leads to diseases such as cancer and heart disease. Some vitamins help detoxify pollutants.

We still have a lot to learn about the role of vitamins in the body. Until we know all that vitamins do and measure all their effects, we really don't know how much of each vitamin we need.

We do know how much can be too much and how much keeps the average healthy person in average health. You, yourself, can find out what the right amount is for you by following the New Supernutrition Plan in this book.

Minerals are more than the structural components of our bones and tissues. Minerals also form parts of enzymes that regulate body chemistry. The B vitamins that help make up the structure of so many enzymes are not much good without the magnesium or zinc also needed for many of those same enzymes. Minerals are needed for the heart to beat, red blood cells to carry oxygen, and enzymes to protect tissues and detoxify pollutants.

As you wouldn't want to build your home or your car with missing or insufficient materials, you don't want to build an inferior body by skimping on minerals.

You don't have to make every meal a balanced meal. However, each day you should get a balance of proteins to get all the building blocks for tissue and enzymes. During the day you should get a balance of fats and carbohydrates. You should also get all the recommended amounts of vitamins and minerals every day. There are exceptions, and some vitamins are stored in the body longer than others. You certainly would want to get enough of all the vitamins and minerals within two days at least. You will feel better and have less chance for illness if you get your recommended amounts every day.

For best health you must get the right amount of vitamins and minerals every day. Vitamins and minerals are nutrients that must be obtained from your diet—except for vitamin D, which can be obtained via sunlight exposure.

Vitamins A, E, and K are readily stored. However, they are consumed during normal body metabolism, so they, too, should be supplied daily.

The trick then becomes how to get our vitamins and minerals in the right amounts. Nutritionists are still debating how to balance the "balanced diet." A nutritionist specializing in macronutrition may design a diet having the right balance of saturated fats, unsaturated fats, complex carbohydrates, and refined carbohydrates, only to have a nutritionist specializing in micronutrition point out that the so-called balanced diet is deficient in chromium, zinc, magnesium, vitamin E, etc.

Even if all nutritionists agreed on what a balanced diet was, real people choose not to eat what they know they should. It is true that we are overfed and undernourished. We may be food-smart, but we eat dumb. We tend to be a lot of talk with little nutrition action.

Smart People Take Supplements

Government surveys always show that highly educated people take more food supplements than the least educated. Regardless if they are seeking nutritional insurance, trying to balance a less-than-perfect diet, or striving for optimal nutrition and superhealth, smart people take supplements. (There are also studies that show that children taking supplements become smarter than those not taking supplements, but that's another story.)

The July 18, 1989 statistics from the National Center for Health Sciences showed that taking supplements was an everyday practice for the better educated. The HANES survey taken in 1974, just prior to the publication of *Supernutrition*, found that 23% of American adults took daily supplements. During 1986 36% of American adults took daily nonprescription supplements.

Moderation

Small deficiencies in trace nutrients can lead to diseases other than the frank nutritional diseases. Cancer, heart disease, and accelerated aging may result from vitamin and mineral deficiencies.

Body chemistry is very complex. Several regulatory mechanisms maintain its chemical balance. The regulators adjust for changing conditions, including most dietary changes. In essence, if we eat balanced meals containing all of the food factors that we need in the appropriate amounts, then body chemistry is normal. However, if our diet gets out of balance, and we eat too much of some components and not enough of other components, body chemistry and blood chemistry get out of whack because the regulatory systems are impaired.

The real culprits that induce disease and aging are not the habits, but the changes in body chemistry that occur when the regulatory system is taxed beyond its capacity. Those changes can be manipulated by several factors.

While the conventional approach attempts to avoid overtaxing the capacity of our regulatory mechanisms, the alternative approach seeks to increase those capacities. If you cannot or will not adjust your life-style, then you should at least fortify your body to withstand your life-style as well as you can.

A "prudent" life-style helps maintain your regulatory systems by reducing the amount of compensation required by your body chemistry, but it can't compensate when the necessary nutrients are lacking.

Smoking, excessive drinking, lack of sleep, inactivity, and even the oversupply of certain food components such as fats put excessive stress on the body. However, if your regulatory systems have an adequate supply of vital nutrients, your normal body chemistry can withstand a great deal of abuse.

There is much virtue in moderation. Religions have preached moderation, and those religions having significant compliance with moderate life-styles are known for their excellent health and longevity. Seventh-Day Adventists and Mormons are examples of those obtaining above-average health and longevity through moderation of life-style.

One epidemiologist, Dr. James Enstrom of the University of California at Los Angeles, has studied Mormon and Seventh-Day Adventist life-styles extensively over many years. I have followed Dr. Enstrom's research closely, and I had the honor of conducting a study with Dr. Linus Pauling and Dr. Enstrom.[1]

In a 1989 study of 10,000 Mormons Dr. Enstrom found that three common factors contributed to their better health and longer life.[2] Middle-aged male Mormons who adhered to the three factors had only 14% of the heart-disease death rate of non-Mormon men of the same age. They also had only 34% of the cancer death rate, and 32% of the overall death rate.

The average life expectancy for a twenty-five-year-old Mormon man is eighty-five years; for other U.S. men, seventy-four. For Mormon women, eighty-six; other U.S. women, eighty.

What are the three factors? Regular physical activity, regular sleep habits, and nonsmoking.

Vegetarianism was not a factor. These religious groups do not advocate vegetarianism, but they eat moderately and include ample fruits and vegetables in their diet. There are many Mormons in Utah, and Utah has the highest per capita consumption of meat.

The word "vegetarian" is not magic. Some who claim "not to eat red meat" or who "don't eat meat at all" actually exist on junk food. They avoid hot dogs and hamburgers but eat doughnuts with coffee for breakfast, peanut butter and jelly sandwiches with soda for lunch, and pizza with beer for dinner. They still eat few vegetables and fruits. There can be so-called "vegetarian" junk diets that are just as unhealthy as standard omnivore junk diets.

But vegetarianism or near-vegetarianism has much to offer to many. Consider the following generalizations:

1. Most vegetarian diets are good diets. They are rich in vitamins, minerals, and fiber. They are moderate in calories, and low in fat and salt.
2. Most non-vegetarian diets are not good diets. They are high in calories, fat, and salt. They are low in vitamins, minerals, and fiber.
3. Vegetarian diets are not efficiently digested, which is fine when there is not a food shortage.

4. Non-vegetarian diets are usually efficiently digested, which is important when there are food shortages.
5. No one diet is best for everyone. Genetic factors influence our ability to tolerate and digest foods and to extract nutrients. Usually, an Eskimo will do better on an Eskimo diet than on an African diet, and vice versa. Germanic descendants may do better on a "meat and potato" diet than on an Italian pasta diet, and vice versa. However, these generalizations are only true if all of the diets are balanced diets.
6. Vegetarians are usually health-conscious, moderate-life-style persons. This is a very healthy life-style combination.
7. Non-vegetarians should strive to add more fruits and vegetables to their diets at the expense of high-fat foods or excess meats. Limiting meats to five to six ounces daily is a reasonable goal for the "average" person of 165 pounds. Some may do better with less, some may do better with more.
8. You can achieve optimal results with a non-vegetarian diet if you balance it correctly. Just do not eat the "Standard American Diet (SAD)." However, you can also achieve optimal results with a vegetarian diet with the use of supplements.

For those who insist on burning it at both ends, let's consider more of the evidence that shows that Mom was right all along.

In 1972 Dr. Lester Breslow and his associates at the University of California reported on a study of the habits of Californians.[3] The Alameda Study found that people who get adequate sleep, eat breakfast, stay lean, avoid empty-calorie snacks, exercise regularly, abstain from or go easy on alcohol, and don't smoke are rewarded with superior health.

Dr. Breslow remarked, "The physical health of men in their mid-fifties who follow six or seven of the (above listed) good health habits is about the same as men twenty years younger who follow three or fewer of the good habits. For men sixty-five to seventy-four who have followed all seven good health habits, the likelihood of dying is about the same as men forty-five to fifty-four who ignored most of these practices.

"Those who followed all of the good practices were in better health at every age than those who followed few."

The study found that income was not a factor, only the number of the good habits followed. A follow-up study showed the increase in life expectancy persisted and was not due to any experimental or study artifact.

A consequence of not knowing about the role of the newer nutrients in health is that many people are suboptimally nourished and thus have somewhat impaired regulatory systems. Few people have perfect health habits; most people abuse themselves to some degree, and their regulatory systems are not able to compensate fully. While prudent measures tend to reduce the amount of abuse your body receives, your body can still receive enough abuse to be harmed. Thus you will have better health with a fully functioning body receiving moderate abuse than with an impaired body receiving only a little abuse. Smokers who are well nourished with vitamin A, for example, have less cancer than malnourished nonsmokers who occasionally breathe air polluted by smokers or factories. Similar studies have been made that indicate that well-nourished moderate drinkers tolerate alcohol better than malnourished occasional drinkers.

The same is true concerning fat intake. We hear so much about the need to reduce our fat intake—which is a good idea. But the fact is that people eating a high-fat diet who are adequately nourished with vitamin C and minerals such as copper have lower blood-cholesterol levels than people on a low-fat diet who are not getting enough copper and vitamin C.

Within limits, either lowered fat intake or increased vitamin E intake will bring about the same improvement in blood chemistry, and either decreasing the amount of sugar in the diet or increasing the amount of a nutrient called carnitine will lower undesirable blood chemicals called triglycerides.

If you are well nourished and follow good habits, you'll enjoy the best health protection. But for the average person who neither is optimally nourished nor has healthy habits, it is easier to optimize nutrition than to quit bad habits, although many people can moderate them. Three-pack-a-day smokers can reduce their smoking by half or even to a pack a day. The sedentary person can learn to enjoy short walks two or three times a week. This is a reasonable "first goal" for these persons. The unmistaken feeling of better health then becomes a driving force for further improvements in health habits.

Serious abuse—four packs a day and twelve drinks a day—will overwhelm the regulatory system no matter how well nourished one is. The alternative strategy presented in this book will offer some protection to those who insist on seriously abusing their bodies but will not protect to the same extent as for the prudent, average-nourished person.

The "alternative" practices discussed in this book control body chemistry more directly and therefore more effectively than many so-called "prudent" practices. And the "alternatives" are easier because they simply involve adding nutrients to our diets rather than denying ourselves the foods we like and forcing ourselves to do exercises that we don't enjoy.

Let's look at the specific ways that vitamins and minerals affect how we age.

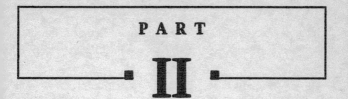

PART

II

Supernutrition Against Aging

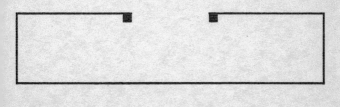

5

Slowing the Aging Process

If you are burning the candle at both ends, here's how you can put more wax in the middle. You can maintain the prime of life longer by applying the discoveries discussed in this chapter.

The extra years you can gain will be the prime-of-life middle years, not extended old age. This chapter will help you revitalize your prime years between thirty and eighty. It is true that we are living longer. And there is no use living longer if you have to sacrifice too much. There is truth in the old joke that some things don't really add years to your life—they only make it seem longer.

Why spend fifteen years of jogging time to add five years to your life span? That's a loss of ten years! Why eat tasteless meals the rest of your life and make eating a chore rather than a pleasure to live five more years of crippled, senile senescence? Is this really a benefit to you or your family? You can live better and an average of fifteen years longer without changing your life-style appreciably.

Slower aging means better skin with fewer wrinkles, a better memory with no senility, no arthritis, and no cataracts. The fact that someone is older in years is no reason for him or her to have diminished sexual fulfillment or to have crippling diseases such as arthritis.

Background

On October 23, 1970, I described my research to the 23rd Annual International Gerontology Conference in Toronto.[1,2] News summaries were published in the scientific press[3] and the lay press.[4,5] My experiments showed that certain combinations of antioxidant nutrients extend the average life span of laboratory animals by 20% to 30% and their maximum life span by 5% to 10%. In experiments designed to accelerate the aging process, antioxidants increased animal life spans by 175% over the shortened life spans of the control animals not receiving the extra antioxidants.

The latter experiments really examined accelerated aging rather than natural life span. The great advantage obtained between the animals protected by the antioxidants is due to their protective effect against life-shortening processes. This is different than extending a normal life span. However, this has meaningful application to real life. We need protection against things that shorten life more than we need something to lengthen our life spans. (I will discuss the new research involving the good news about extending the *maximum* life span later.)

We are currently living an average life span of seventy-five years, with some individuals living over one hundred. Projections that I made in the 1960s indicate that our natural average life span should be eighty-five years, with a number of persons living to 115 years.

Optimal nourishment will help many get an extra five or ten years over the average, but the greatest benefit in life-extension will be for the multitudes of people who are shortening their lives with undernourishment and bad habits. Antioxidant undernourishment will make you older than your years.

Keep in mind that the extra five or ten years is not as important as the extra ten to fifteen years of improved health. Remember, the goal is not to live longer, but to live *better* longer.

Antioxidant Nutrients and Free Radicals

As *Supernutrition* stated, the keys to slowing aging with optimal nutrition are antioxidant nutrients. The primary antioxidant nutrients are vitamin A and beta-carotene, vitamin C, vitamin E, and the trace mineral selenium. These nutrients are called "antioxidants" because they prevent body components from destruction by oxygen. Chemical reactions with oxygen power the body. However, sometimes oxygen reacts with body components in undesirable ways.

Antioxidant nutrients combine with oxygen more easily than the components that they are designed to protect. Thus, antioxidant nutrients sacrifice themselves to oxygen to save delicate cell membranes and other vital body components. Antioxidant nutrients help the desired reactions with oxygen to proceed normally on controlled pathways while preventing the undesired reactions from occurring.

Now we have new antioxidants such as Pycnogenol and beta-carotene to extend the synergism. They will be listed later in the "Supplements" section of this chapter.

Other researchers, such as Dr. Denham Harman of the University of Nebraska School of Medicine, England's Dr. Alex Comfort, and Dr. Al Tappel of the University of California at Davis, have found that individual antioxidant nutrients produce significant life span increases. However, the additive effect of the individual nutrients is less than that of the synergistic combinations of antioxidant nutrients.

Dr. Harman was the originator of the free-radical theory of aging.[6] However, in his experiments using single antioxidants, the life-span improvements were not dramatic, and the quantities that were required to be effective would be impractical for human use at levels approaching 5% of the total diet. My synergistic quantities bring about dramatic life-span increases and only require a few grams of antioxidants, which are not only safe and effective, but within the "megavitamin" range used by so many now.

My research was not a follow-up of Dr. Harman's research. In 1963, when I was a laboratory director for Allied Chemical Corporation, a portion of my work involved oxidation reactions involving elements such as oxygen, chlorine, and fluorine. My research involved industrial materials, but personally, I was also interested in oxidation problems in the body that led to deteriorated performance. I was especially interested in why an athlete becomes slower with age, in spite of continual conditioning.

I was also interested in the protective effect of vitamin E in maintaining athletic performance. I found that vitamin E protected athletic performance by protecting tissues and organs against excessive oxidation. More recent research on this subject measured breakdown products (such as pentane) in expelled breath and found that exercise increases the need for vitamin E.[7] This extra need for vitamin E has been confirmed by measuring other cellular compounds.[8–10]

In 1963 my experiments involved "test tube"–type studies of antioxidants for protection against "cross-linking." Cross-linking is the deleterious joining together of two molecules so that the action of each is impaired. It's like welding or handcuffing the molecules together.

I began by using ultraviolet radiation to initiate cross-linking of polyunsaturated fatty acids in a gelatin matrix. The protective action of the antioxidants could be measured by determining the amount of polymerization or cross-linking of the gelatin by gas chromatography and melting-point studies.

In 1966 I started small-scale studies using laboratory animals to determine if the combinations of antioxidants that were synergistic in the test-tube studies were also biologically synergistic in mammalians.

Another researcher, Dr. Johan Bjorksten, was also researching this area at the time. Dr. Bjorksten was studying which compounds caused cross-linking.[11] He was also looking for an enzyme that would undo cross-linking. As it turned out, in attempting to use ultraviolet energy to produce cross-linkages in fats distributed in gelatin in my laboratory, I found that antioxidants prevented cross-linking, and that certain combinations in certain proportions were synergistic. Literature research on antioxidants then led me to the research of Drs. Harman and Tappel. Later I confirmed that free radicals can cause cross-linking, and that direct chemical reactions can cause cross-linking.

Dr. Tappel was the first to confirm that my mixture was synergistic. He found that my formula was more than twice as protective as could be estimated from the additive effects alone.[12] My research also showed that this synergism protects against cancer.[13]

Antioxidants will help protect you against the damage that adds signs of aging to your body, and they will add a few years of life. It doesn't mean that antioxidants will reverse aging or double your life span. It means that you can have the health and body of a person many years younger than you.

Antioxidants also work chemically by blocking free-radical reactions that do not involve oxygen. The December 1971 issue of *Prevention* magazine was the first lay magazine to discuss my research and report on free radicals to the general public.[5]

Free radicals are highly reactive, unstable compounds or molecular fragments that will react with just about anything. They are chemical terrorists! They can be generated in the body and have the potential to do great harm to body cells. (A more detailed description of free radicals appears on page 40.) Free-radical chemistry is an important theme in this book. It is the key to slowing aging and preventing cancer, heart disease, and arthritis.

Free radicals alter cell membranes in such a way as to kill the cell or change it to a cancer cell. Free radicals can also bind compounds together in such a way as to alter their function or the physical characteristics of the entire tissue. As an example, young, babylike skin can be made as tough as leather by the actions of free radicals produced by sunlight.

Rather than bore you with an entire chapter on free-radical chemistry, I will present a little at a time in several chapters.

In addition to longer life spans of laboratory animals receiving adequate amounts of antioxidant nutrients, further studies showed that these nutrients dramatically reduced the incidence of cancer. This was true even when the animals were fed chemicals that cause cancer or were injected with cancer cells.

This information was available to readers of my earlier books, such as *Supernutrition* in 1975 and *Cancer and Its Nutritional Therapies* in 1978. Now there is fifteen years' worth of additional research to help you live better longer and to be freer of the risk of the major killer diseases longer.

Before discussing this new research, let's look at the aging process itself.

FREE RADICALS

■   ■

Free radicals are unstable, highly reactive compounds or molecular fragments. Compounds consist of two or more elements held together by a chemical attraction called a "bond." The bonding involves negatively charged parts of the atoms called "electrons." The arrangement of the electrons determines the stability of the compound.

A stable compound has electrons that are in pairs. It's like a buddy system. It is a state of lower energy as the electrons spin in opposite directions. In nature, all systems seek the lowest energy level. However, if an electron is not paired with another, it becomes very reactive and unstable. It will seek out another electron to pair with. In the process of grabbing a partner, a reaction between compounds occurs, and the other compound can become a free radical and perpetuate the process. One free radical can damage a million or more molecules by this self-perpetuating process. The process can be stopped by compounds called "free-radical scavengers." Most antioxidants are good free-radical scavengers.

Do not confuse free radicals with ions. Ions are formed when electrons are removed and an electrical imbalance results in the atom or molecule having a positive or negative charge. Neutral atoms and molecules can be free radicals, as can ions.

What Is Aging?

There is no one physical or mental condition directly attributed simply to the passage of time. Some of the alleged diseases of aging—such as high blood pressure and arthritis—are prevalent in the very young as well as the very old. What exactly is aging, then, and what are its causes?

Aging is the process that reduces the number of healthy cells in the body. The most striking factor in the aging process is the body's loss of reserves due to the decreasing number of cells in each organ. For example, fasting blood glucose (sugar) levels remain fairly constant throughout life, but the glucose-tolerance measurement shows a loss of response in aging. Glucose tolerance measures the *reserve* capacity of this system to respond to the stress of the glucose load. The same holds true for the recovery mechanisms of other systems.

Slowing the Aging Process

Free-radical reactions result in the body's loss of active cells. The cumulative effect of billions of cellular free-radical reactions is to add to the body's loss of reserves. Thus, if we decrease the number of free radicals by increasing the amount of antioxidant nutrients in the body, we slow aging.

There are five main ways in which free radicals age the body.

(1) Lipid peroxidation, in which free radicals damage fatty compounds, causing them to turn rancid and to release more free radicals in a chain reaction.

(2) Cross-linking, in which free radicals cause proteins and DNA to fuse together. DNA is the substance that replicates the body components. It's the protein factory that can reproduce itself or whatever the body needs. Altered DNA can't make what the body needs. Instead, useless debris is formed, which clogs the body's mechanisms.

(3) Membrane damage, in which free radicals destroy the integrity of cell membranes. This interferes with the cells' ability to absorb nutrients and expel waste products. Both events kill cells.

(4) Lysosomal damage, in which free radicals rupture lysosome membranes. Lysosomes are enzymes that can digest just about anything except the membranes that store them. When the membrane sac that stores them is ruptured by free radicals, the lysosomes spill into the cell interior and destroy critical parts. The cell dies and becomes another clinker or burned-out light bulb in the marquee of life.

(5) Miscellaneous free-radical reactions form residues called lipofuscin or age pigment. These residues accumulate with time and interfere with cell function and the life processes.

My research in slowing the aging process involves more than preventing damage by slowing free-radical reactions. The damage caused by free radicals can continue to age the body by tying up needed components such as DNA. Also, body compounds that are misproduced can cause immunological reactions that hasten aging. The damage that has occurred from free-radical reactions must be *undone* if appreciable life extension is to occur. The body has repair enzymes such as macroxyproteinase and phospholipases that can undo part of the damage.

A brief description of my unifying theory of free-radical aging can be found on page 43.

Without a means of stimulating and maintaining the health of the "repair" enzymes, my progress so far has been to show a "secondary effect" on the aging process rather than to slow the "primary cause" of aging. Slowing the secondary effects produces the modest gain of five to ten years of healthy life, reduces the risk of major diseases, and protects against premature aging.

The applicable antioxidant nutrients and their effective intakes are listed in Table 5.1, page 48.

New Research

A new and more powerful antioxidant nutrient has been discovered. "Pycnogenol" is the trade name for a patented mixture of oligomeric and monomeric proanthocyanidins. Proanthocyanidins are members of the bioflavonoid family of compounds. Pycnogenol can be extracted from grape seeds and vines, but the commercial source is normally the bark of the French maritime pine (*Pinus pinaster* or *Pinus maritime*).

This powerful antioxidant has been tested for safety at the Pasteur Institute and Huntington Institute. European researchers have found that Pycnogenol is important to artery and skin health; but more importantly, Pycnogenol is a proven free-radical scavenger. Pycnogenol is fifty times better than vitamin E and twenty times better than vitamin C against free radicals.

As stated earlier, the *maximum* life span is the best measure of the aging rate. My antioxidant nutrients significantly

FREE-RADICAL AGING

Briefly, my unified theory of aging was assembled from my own research on blocking cross-linking, protein missynthesis resorters, excitation of double bonds, and singlet oxygen, plus the research of other gerontologists. The theory focuses on alterations of DNA and RNA by free-radical reactions initiated by radiation or oxygen (both triplet and singlet). Free radicals cause proteins—particularly enzymes—to be synthesized incorrectly, leading to the death of cells. Antioxidant nutrients terminate free-radical chain reactions. Selenium compounds help break up incorrectly synthesized proteins through disulfide linkages. Disulfide bonds and double bonds are exposed for an abnormally long period during changes in conformation and are electromagnetically influenced by selenium bonds.[14-18]

extended *average* life span and had a small effect on the *maximum* life span. Thus, the antioxidants that I used had a secondary effect on the aging process but did not slow the primary aging process.

The question is whether this life extension is due to much-improved heart health and strengthened immunity or to slowing the primary aging process.

In 1981 Dr. Emile Bliznakov, scientific director of the Lupus Research Institute in Ridgefield, Connecticut, reported that he had extended the maximum life span of mice with the nutrient Coenzyme Q-10 (CoQ-10). This is a new nutrient to most people.

Our ability to make this important compound seems to decrease as we age. In some people, their ability to make CoQ-10 becomes so impaired that they depend almost entirely on their diet for their CoQ-10. In such cases, CoQ-10 can be said to assume vitamin status. CoQ-10 can be found in many fresh foods, but it is a fragile compound that is easily destroyed by oxidation, processing, and cooking. Organ meats, spinach, whole grains, beef, sardines, peanuts, nuts, and seeds are good sources of CoQ-10 or its precursors.

Dr. Bliznakov divided a large number of old white laboratory mice into two equal smaller groups. The groups were fed and treated the same, except the "experimental" group was also given CoQ-10. All mice in the "control" group (not fed the CoQ-10) died of natural causes within nine months of the start of the experiment. The mice were about seventeen months old at the start of the experiment, which is equivalent to a human age of about sixty-eight years. The life spans of the control group were normal for that species.

The experimental group taking CoQ-10 were not all dead until more than *twenty months* after the start of the experiment.[19] To have the strain of mice used in the experiment live for three years is quite an achievement. One immediately has to wonder how long these mice would live if they were given extra CoQ-10 from a very early age.

The CoQ-10 group not only lived more than twice as long after the experiment started as the control group, but *they lived much longer than mice normally do when they live their maximum life span*. This is the difference between extending the average life span and extending the maximum life span.

Not only did the CoQ-10 mice live longer, but they had great vigor and mobility, more lustrous hair, brighter eyes, and absence of the normal signs of advanced age. Three or four of the CoQ-10 mice lived to the equivalent of 130 to 150 years of human life, and yet they still appeared youthful.

Just as humans do, laboratory mice dying in old age normally die of natural causes related to heart failure, cancer, and infections. CoQ-10 could protect against any or all of these afflictions, and/or it could slow the primary aging process.

This experiment is so exciting that more scientists must confirm the experiment and then must investigate the mechanism by which CoQ-10 works. This much is known: CoQ-10 is a very powerful antioxidant and has a very beneficial effect on heart health. (This will be discussed in later chapters.)

At this writing, UCLA gerontologists Drs. Roy Walford and Steven Harris are more than three years into an experiment that can confirm Dr. Bliznakov's results and also further extend our knowledge.

Another new antioxidant that looks very promising is Superoxide Dismutase (SOD). SOD is produced in the body to counteract superoxide free radicals. Gerontologists have shown that the animals of any given species that live longest are those that have the highest SOD levels in their blood.

It has also been shown that SOD production normally tapers off as an individual ages. Liver-based supplements rich in SOD are a source of SOD, although the SOD is poorly absorbed by humans.

SOD is a large molecule, and little is assimilated intact, though studies have shown SOD lasting long enough in the bloodstream to be effective.

However, a better way of increasing your level of SOD may soon be on the way. If experiments by Japanese researcher Dr. Yukie Niwa can be applied to large-scale production methods, SOD activity can be produced in food in such a way as to be readily absorbed. Dr. Niwa has shown that special food preparation based on methods similar to traditional Japanese cooking can split SOD into smaller fragments that retain SOD's ability to counteract the superoxide free radical.

Growth Hormone

Newspaper and TV accounts of a study published in the *New England Journal of Medicine* in July 1990 created quite a stir.[20] The story on Cable News Network showed "little old men" springing along with big smiles and saying that they felt like supermen.

The clinical trial showed that injections of human growth hormone increased muscle mass and decreased body fat. It had other rejuvenating effects that appeared to reverse at least some aspects of the aging process.

Growth hormone secretion declines with age. The hormone does more than regulate growth. It stimulates the immune system and is a factor in repairing the body. Unfortunately, growth hormone injections are very expensive. According to the study, the cost of the hormone alone is $13,000 a year.

However, diet can have an effect on the manufacture and release of growth hormone. An Italian study of twelve men showed that the amino acids arginine and lysine increase growth hormone secretion.[21] Other natural metabolites such as GABA (gamma amino butyric acid) and GHB (gamma hydroxyl butyrate) also cause growth hormone secretion to increase, but they have other undesirable side effects that need to be further studied.

Moderation and Tranquillity

There is more to slowing the aging process than CoQ-10 and antioxidant vitamins and minerals. There is some "prudent" advice that you should consider. Only in this case it doesn't stem from incomplete medical studies, but from the time- (and scientifically) proven wisdom of *Mom*.

Remember the studies about moderation discussed in the preceding chapter? Moderation and a happy, peaceful, active mind are very important.

Another major key to living better longer is happiness. Many, many studies show that happy people live longer. People who have positive attitudes, are satisfied with their lives, help others, sing a lot, laugh a lot, smile a lot, and are involved with people rather than things are healthier and live longer.

Exceptionally long-lived persons tend to live in "today's world," with an eye to the future and little tendency to dwell in the past. They are active, involved, and helpful. Most important, they never cease an activity just because of age. Satchel Paige, who pitched major league baseball in his fifties and possibly his sixties (he would never admit his true age), expressed this concept most eloquently. He simply asked, "How old would you be if you didn't know how old you was?"

Mom's proven "moderation" rules do not involve dietary fat, cholesterol, or fiber—but they do mention smoking, drinking, and exercise. Not to despair! That's what this book is about. Of course, you will be better off if you exercise, don't smoke, and are not an alcoholic. But if you choose to disregard those health rules, or just can't help yourself, then this book will show you how to compensate for those "bad" habits. You can even have better health and a longer life than those who follow all seven of the good health practices but are suboptimally nourished.

While we're talking moderation, let's be moderate in our pursuit of moderation! Life is for living. Let's not abuse ourselves, but let's have fun, too! Being fanatical defeats the purpose of moderation. All that worry would upset your body chemistry and cause great harm over the years. Moderation doesn't mean that you have to give up anything you like—you just use better judgment of when enough is enough. In fact, moderation will give you better health and longer life to *enjoy* doing whatever it is that turns you on.

Supplements

You can increase the flame of life by using the correct fuels—optimal nutrition. Try it—you'll see that you can do more for longer, and really have fun now and years later in your extended prime. You will need no other aphrodisiac.

If you insist on burning the candle at both ends, you can slow the burning and burn more brightly with antioxidant vitamins and minerals. You can put more wax in the middle with the new powerful antioxidant nutrient CoQ-10.

You may wish to consider the following supplements to reduce the rate at which you might otherwise age. The major antioxidant nutrients are Pycnogenol, CoQ-10, vitamins A, C, and E, the trace mineral selenium, and the amino acid cysteine.

Vitamin C is the major antioxidant in the blood. Vitamin C completely protects blood fats against peroxyl free-radical attack.[22] It is the only antioxidant that can do this in the blood. Vitamin C stabilizes the superoxide free radical, stabilizes the hydroxyl free radical, and quenches singlet oxygen.

Vitamin E is the major antioxidant in the cell membrane. Vitamin E protects against lipid peroxidation of cell membranes, stabilizes the superoxide free radical, stabilizes the hydroxyl free radical, and quenches singlet oxygen.

Vitamin A is the major antioxidant in mucous membranes,

TABLE 5.1
Ranges of Supplementation to Slow Aging

Nutrient	Daily Amount
Pycnogenol	50–100 mg
Coenzyme Q-10 (CoQ-10)	15–60 mg
Vitamin A	5,000–15,000 IU
Vitamin C	1,500–10,000 mg
Vitamin E	200–800 IU
Selenium	50–200 mcg
Cysteine	500–1,000 mg
Ascorbyl palmitate (or Ester-C)	as labeled
Beta-carotene	5,000–11,000 IU
Pantothenic acid	250–500 mg
Vitamin B-6	25–50 mg
SOD (superoxide dismutase)	as labeled
Lysine	500–1,000 mg
Methionine	500–1,000 mg
Arginine or ornithine	500–1,000 mg
Glutathione	100–250 mg
Zinc	15–25 mg

and selenium, in the form of glutathione peroxidase, protects the aqueous portions of cells.

The list includes the important new antioxidants Pycnogenol, beta-carotene, ascorbyl palmitate, and glutathione. Ascorbyl palmitate and Ester-C are fat-soluble forms of vitamin C that extend vitamin C protection into fat storage areas, where it protects against free radical reactions called lipid peroxidation. Beta-carotene is the most efficient quencher of singlet oxygen, an unwanted oxygen form that is as harmful as free-radical reactions.

Minor antioxidants are listed in the table as well. The major immune system and human growth hormone stimulants are the amino acids lysine, arginine, and ornithine. The antioxidant vitamins C and E and selenium are also effective immune system stimulants.

You may wish to consider the ranges of supplementation in Table 5.1, or you may wish to change your diet to include foods rich in these nutrients. However, keep in mind that food tables are not accurate concerning selenium, and food tables do not yet include the newly discovered nutrients.

Gastric problems are common in persons over the age of fifty years. Poor digestion affects our ability to extract and absorb nutrients from food. This fact alone makes it prudent to include vitamin and mineral supplements in the diet of middle-aged and older persons.

Remember, the quantities of nutrients suggested are not additive. As an example, if two different chapters recommend the same nutrient, don't add the quantities together. Just be sure to be somewhere in the optimal range.

That's the basic story of slowing the aging process with antioxidant nutrients and CoQ-10. We all can't live to be a hundred years old, but we can live much longer than we would if we didn't protect ourselves from premature aging with supplements and life-style changes. The most important benefit will be the quality of our lives.

The next several chapters contain specific information on preventing wrinkles, memory loss, senility, and cataracts; easing menopause; and preventing prostate and impotence problems. If you have no interest in these specific areas, just jump ahead to Chapter 12 in Section III, which examines how antioxidant nutrients prevent cancer.

6

Younger Skin

Your skin serves several functions, including excretion. Not sweat; that's a cooling function. When the body can't eliminate some toxins fast enough through the kidneys, they are dumped into the skin and hair. These toxins can take the glow out of healthy skin and even cause blemishes. Therefore, be sure that you keep your primary excretion mechanisms working efficiently.

The single most important nutrient for beautiful skin is water! Your daily diet should include the equivalent of six to eight eight-ounce glasses of water. The nutrient of next greatest importance is fiber. The following chapter will discuss fiber in more detail, but general recommendations will be presented shortly. Fiber and the good bacteria such as *Lactobacillus acidophilus* and *Lactobacillus bulgaricus* help eliminate toxins from the bowel that might otherwise be absorbed and "dumped" into the skin.

Vitamin A is also important, along with the mineral zinc, which is required to make the protein that carries vitamin A to the skin. Unsaturated fatty acids such as linolenic and eicosapentaenoic acid (EPA) are critical for supple young skin. Pet owners have seen the difference in skin and hair that adding such oils to their pet's diet makes. It works for us, too.

Not too much—just enough to help oil the skin from the inside. And be sure to take enough vitamins A and E to protect against the oils causing free radicals to form from lipid peroxidation.

Wrinkling

You can choose to use the sun's beneficial rays through moderate exposure, or you can choose to age and wrinkle your skin through overexposure. If you bake in the sun most of the time, you can really ruin your skin—with skin cancer. The ultraviolet energy from the sun produces free radicals in the fats stored in the skin cell membranes. The two greatest sources of free radicals in the skin are sunlight and cigarette smoke.

If you want to test this theory, just examine the skin on the back of the necks of fishermen or farmers and compare this to skin on the same people that has been protected from the sun, such as on their buttocks. You will get wrinkles on your face, neck, and hands before you will on your mostly unexposed parts.

The main protein in skin, collagen, can have its molecules cross-linked or fused together by free radicals. Normal collagen molecules slide over one another. This is the case in young, pliable skin. Collagen molecules fused together make skin tissue rigid and leathery. A test of skin's apparent age is to pinch the skin on the top of the back of your hand and see how fast it returns to its normal position.

The key to delaying wrinkling is to not overexpose yourself to the sun. If you really want to be fanatical about having young-looking skin, just stay out of the sun unless you are wearing a strong sunscreen or sun-blocking agent such as PABA-containing lotions. Also be sure to wear a hat in the sun and to take antioxidant nutrients such as vitamins A, C, and especially E, plus the mineral selenium.

Pycnogenol has been shown to be important in skin health. Dr. R. Kuttan and colleagues have shown that pycnogenol binds tightly to skin collagen and increases its resistance to enzyme degradation.[1] It also helps repair collagen.

In addition to being a good free-radical destroyer, vitamin

C is an important skin nutrient, as it is required in the production of collagen.

Cigarettes are the next leading cause of premature wrinkling. Although the results vary with the number of cigarettes smoked, on average a pack-and-a-half-a-day smoker will wrinkle about ten years sooner than a nonsmoker.

The same free-radical fighters mentioned above will reduce the wrinkling action of smoking.

Good nutrition and a good moisturizer will help maintain skin moisture and reduce wear and tear. Moisturizers are constantly being improved through research, but the best at this writing seems to be the sodium salt of pyrollidone carboxylic acid, which is abbreviated on labels as NaPCA. NaPCA is abundant in young skin, but sparse in aged skin. You may wish to look for NaPCA on the label the next time you buy a moisturizer, but there are many good products out there, and you should find the one best for your skin. Using any natural oil is better than not using any moisturizer.

Don't forget a sunscreen after bathing.

Supplements

Consult Table 6.1 for nutrients that you may wish to consider as part of your dietary skin care. Smokers may wish to take other nutrients as well—L-cysteine, for example.

TABLE 6.1
Skin Care Nutrients

Nutrient	Daily Amount
Water	6–8 8-oz. glasses
Fiber	enough to ensure that your stools float
Pycnogenol	50–150 mg
Beta-carotene	5,000–11,000 IU
Vitamin A	5,000–10,000 IU
Vitamin C	250–1,000 mg
Vitamin E	50–400 IU
Selenium	50–200 mcg
PABA	25–150 mg
Linolenic acid	as labeled
Eicosapentaenoic acid (EPA)	as labeled
Gamma-linolenic acid (GLA)	as labeled
Lactobacillus acidophilus (or *L. bulgaricus* from yogurt)	as labeled

7

Memory, Senility, and Alzheimer's

■

There are several food supplements that improve your memory, but I forget what they are. Of course, it is normal to momentarily forget things, but when we get older, we worry about becoming senile. Now we have evidence that dietary supplements can improve the memory of the young and old alike and even alleviate some types of senility.

The ability of brain neurons (nerve cells) to make and release several of their neurotransmitters (compounds that carry the nerve impulse from one neuron to another) depends directly on the concentration of amino acids in the blood, and therefore on the most recent meal. The brain is unable to make sufficient quantities of amino acids and choline to satisfy its need for neurotransmitter production. The brain must therefore obtain these precursor molecules from the general blood supply.

Each meal can modify blood amino acid and choline contents, alter brain L-tryptophan (see Chapter 9) and choline levels, and thereby affect the rate at which neurons produce the neurotransmitters serotonin and acetylcholine respectively.

Many research teams are studying means to use the brain's dependence on dietary nutrients to learn more about brain function as well as to treat states thought to result from inadequate release of nutrient-dependent neurotransmitters. Examples of such diseases include tardive dyskinesia (involuntary, repetitive movements of the lower face), Huntington's disease (an inherited disease that causes progressive degeneration of the brain), and Alzheimer's disease (a progressive degeneration of the brain not linked to heredity).

Choline and Normal Memory

Researchers were astonished to find that the key neurotransmitter, acetylcholine, was so dependent on diet. Acetylcholine is made when a molecule of choline joins a molecule of acetylcoenzyme A via an enzymatic reaction. However, this enzyme is not very efficient and is very dependent on how much choline is present. Acetylcholine concentrations rise within all neurons inside and outside of the brain, and in the nerve terminal from which the neurotransmitter is released to go to the next nerve cell.

Further research has shown that blood choline levels in humans normally vary as a function of dietary choline content, and that the dietary constituent lecithin provides choline more efficiently to the brain than does the free-form dietary choline itself. Further research has determined that a more efficient ingredient in lecithin for supplying choline to the brain is phosphatidyl choline, which is available as a dietary supplement.

Furthermore, the studies of one researcher, Dr. Ronald Mervis of Ohio State University, indicate that a form of lecithin is particularly effective in preventing nerve damage. The lecithin is an oil-free lecithin powder containing 95% phosphatides. It is rich in phosphatidyl choline, phosphatidylethanolamine, and phosphatidyl inositol.

Typical studies involving choline and memory have included showing that high doses of choline significantly enhanced the ability of college students to recall lengthy word sequences, an animal study showing choline prevented the decline in memory normally associated with age, and another that demonstrated that the brain cells themselves were protected from deterioration by dietary supplementation.

In one study of persons aged twenty-one to twenty-nine it was found that choline taken ninety minutes before a test of nonrelated word recall enhanced all recall in those subjects over those taking an inert placebo, but what was particularly interesting was that the ability to recall abstract words was enhanced the most. The recall of highly imageable words such as "train" and "hat" was considerably enhanced, but the recall of poorly imageable words such as "truth" and "justice" was greatly enhanced. This suggests that there may be two routes of memorization, one involving visualization and the other not, with choline playing an important part in the abstract memory.

So it has been shown that dietary supplements can increase brain function and memory in the young and old alike. But I shouldn't say "alike," because the effect becomes more pronounced with age. Aging damages the brain cells, largely through free-radical reactions. The antioxidant nutrients will slow this damage, but if it has already occurred, then dietary nutrients such as choline and lecithin can help compensate for the damage.

Nerve cells in young people are long, with many branches (dendrites). The dendrites act like antennas in a communications network to receive messages from other nerve cells. However, as we age we lose many of these dendrites, and our nerve transmissions suffer. Messages don't go through, or they are shorted out.

Also as we age, we lose efficency in producing acetylcholine. The sluggish enzyme involved in acetylcholine production needs more help. But even more distressing is that the enzyme that destroys acetylcholine increases in quantity as we age. If this isn't enough, the receptors that catch acetylcholine lose some of their ability to capture it as we age. Thus we need more and more choline-supplying nutrients as we age to maintain maximum brain function and memory.

In one promising experiment, middle-aged mice fed a high-choline diet had the memories of young mice, while other middle-aged mice fed a low-choline diet had the poor memory function of aged mice.

B-Complex Vitamins and Memory

Recent studies show that a small but significant percentage of patients institutionalized in nursing homes or state hospitals for senility or psychosis actually have vitamin B-12 deficiency. Dr. James S. Goodwin of the University of New Mexico School of Medicine in Albuquerque is a leader in memory research in the elderly who recommends that all patients with memory problems or mental symptoms be tested for vitamin B-12 deficiency.

Vitamin B-1 should also be considered in treating alcoholics for memory disorders. Alcoholics usually become vitamin B-1 deficient, which leads to many problems, including Wernicke-Korsakoff syndrome, a disease in which victims confabulate, answering questions regardless of fact. These individuals have almost no ability to remember recent events. They cannot learn anything new and have no idea they even have a problem.

A deficiency in another member of the vitamin B complex seems to be involved in memory problems, but the supporting studies so far have not been "placebo controlled." However, it appears that changing the diets of those committed to institutions because of memory disorders results in shorter stays if the patients receive folic acid supplements.

Glutamine and Memory

Another factor involved in brain function and memory is energy level. Brain activity requires more energy than most people realize. The brain has a very high metabolic rate and requires a disproportionate percentage (20%) of the total heart blood output to provide it with sufficient amounts of oxygen and fuel. Most scientists translate "brain fuel" to mean blood sugar (glucose). They tend to forget that the brain also burns glutamic acid as fuel.

The most efficient way to increase the glutamic acid content of the brain—and thus its energy level—is to provide adequate quantities of the amino acid L-glutamine in the diet. L-glutamine is transported through the brain-blood barrier efficiently, whereas glutamic acid is not. Brain cells can convert the L-glutamine into glutamic acid and then convert the glutamic acid into energy for brain function.

Many people suffer from low blood sugar or hypoglycemia and thus have limited blood sugar to fuel the brain. This is why they become confused and irritable during low-blood-sugar attacks. The brain can be kept on high power with extra L-glutamine in the diet regardless of the ups and downs of the blood-sugar level.

Good results have also been obtained with L-glutamate, and further clinical trials are continuing.[1]

Boron and Brain Function

Volunteers on low-boron diets have changes in the electrical impulses that seem to correlate with mental alertness. The study by Drs. James G. Penland and Forrest Nielsen and colleagues correlates well with previous animal studies.

Boron is a mineral that at this time has not been proven to be essential in humans. However, with the new findings reported here and in other chapters, it seems that it is only a matter of time until boron is recognized as essential.

The electrical impulse changes also indicate that a boron deficiency can cause different regions in the brain to get out of sync. Supplementation with three milligrams of boron daily restored the brain's electrical impulses to normal.

Preventing Senility

This section elaborates on the prevention of senility. If this is of no concern to you, then please skip on to the next section that interests you.

As youths, we envisioned the elderly as mostly senile. We feared that we would grow old and senile. The good news is that gerontologists have found that senility is far more rare than we were led to believe. In 1980, only about 11% of the population over age sixty-five showed some form of dementia, the medical term for senility. Less than 5% of our senior citizens actually were severely demented, and nearly two thirds of these patients had Alzheimer's disease.

The situation becomes more grave for those over eighty years of age. Alzheimer's disease may affect 20% of the very aged.

Dementia is not a single disease. The elderly exhibit many of the same types of organic brain syndromes as younger persons (for example, trauma, tumors, alcohol and drug intoxication, infections, and certain hereditary diseases). The several types of mental disorders due to hardening of the arteries or nerve degeneration occur overwhelmingly in the aged, however.

Alzheimer's disease, though, is a growing problem. The disease was called "presenile dementia" by German pathologist Dr. Alois Alzheimer (1864–1915). However, modern research has identified Alzheimer's disease as markedly similar to the senile dementia that affects most of the 5% of the elderly.

Progressive, irreversible dementia will destroy the patient's ability to function in society. The daily life of sufferers becomes a series of overwhelming challenges as they struggle to recognize others or remember how to feed themselves. Death usually follows within seven to ten years of diagnosis.

The changes most commonly associated with Alzheimer's disease occur in the proteins of the nerve cells of the cerebral cortex—the outer layer of the brain—leading to an accumulation of neurofibrillary tangles. These threadlike jumbles of filaments are often found in association with memory loss, disorientation, and intellectual and other symptoms in patients with Alzheimer's disease. However, tangles are observed in limited quantities in the nerve cells of more than half of the elderly.

Another difference in the Alzheimer's disease patient's brain is in the large number of neuritic plaques from disintegrating nerve cells. There are several biochemical differences as well. Sugar (glucose) metabolism is altered, and at least two neurotransmitters are extremely deficient in the Alzheimer's disease patient's brain. It is hoped that the dietary supplementation of the precursors for these neurotransmitters will be of some value. At this writing, early trials are producing mixed results.

As discussed in the previous section on memory, the brain fuel glutamic acid can be increased by taking L-glutamine. L-glutamine is carried through the brain-blood barrier into brain cells, where it is converted to glutamic acid, a secondary brain fuel.

Aluminum and Alzheimer's Disease

Still another chemical difference may be of importance. In the 1970s a University of Toronto study found aluminum concentration ten to 30 times above normal in the brains of Alzheimer's disease patients.[2] Injection of aluminum into rabbits has produced aluminum-containing neurofibrillary tangles in their brains, but the tangles appear to be different.

A study granted by the British government correlates the incidence of Alzheimer's disease with the amount of aluminum in drinking water.[3,4] The incidence of Alzheimer's disease was 50% higher in areas where there were high concentrations of aluminum in the water, compared to those in low-aluminum areas.

In 1990, Dr. Harvey Singer of the Johns Hopkins School of Medicine found that aluminum produces the same changes in nerve cells that are found in Alzheimer's patients. He reminded us that much more evidence would be needed to establish a definite link, but "it lends further support to the notion that aluminum is a neurotoxin."

There are many dietary sources of aluminum. The amount of aluminum in water is comparatively small, but it is all in solution and ready for absorption into the body. Aluminum is an anti-caking agent used in many flours, is added to table salt to keep it free-flowing, and is a component of many antacids. These forms of aluminum may not be very soluble except under acid conditions, whereas aluminum in water is already solubilized.

There is considerable similarity between early Alzheimer's stages and the encephalopathy induced by aluminum in kidney dialysis patients.

The data are too fragmentary at this time to draw a scientific conclusion. Also, peer review has pointed out areas of possible flaws in the study. However, if future studies do implicate dietary aluminum, drugs can be devised that could chelate out the aluminum from the brain.

Still, the possibility remains that in Alzheimer's disease the neural cell metabolism is progressively impaired by a combination of aluminum excess and lack of essential trace elements.[5]

Choline and Alzheimer's Disease

Choline levels seem to decrease with age in the general population. Alzheimer's disease is linked to impaired function of brain acetylcholine. As mentioned earlier, brain choline is improved by supplementation with phosphatidyl choline or lecithin. One small clinical trial with eleven Alzheimer's disease patients found that seven patients experienced significant improvement in long-term memory. The degree of the memory improved ranged from 50% to 200%.[6]

Antioxidant Nutrients and Alzheimer's Disease

A body of literature is growing to indicate that antioxidant nutrients may help protect against Alzheimer's disease. Unfortunately, this knowledge is of little value to those already afflicted.

Vitamin E deficiency may lower the age of onset and escalate the rate of progression of Alzheimer's disease, according to the conclusions of researchers at the Institute of Psychiatry and Maudsley Hospital in London. They found that 60% of their Alzheimer's patients were deficient in vitamin E. The patients averaged a vitamin E intake of only one third the RDA, and their blood levels of vitamin E were below normal standards.[7]

Researchers have suggested that free-radical attack on

brain cells can affect brain function.[8] They have confirmed that dietary supplements can increase the levels of vitamin E and selenium in brain tissue and thus "provide maintenance of normal, active brain function."

Experimental Supplements Under Study

From fragmentary, uncontrolled, "anecdotal" types of clinical experiences, there does seem to be limited hope for the occasional senile patient. This information is reported here to add to your knowledge in case you feel that it might be worth a try in the case of someone dear to you. As with any experimental program, you and your physician must be exceptionally alert for any undesirable side effects.

TABLE 7.1
Supplements to Prevent Senility

Nutrient	Daily Amount
Choline	500–1,000 mg
Lecithin	as labeled
Phosphatidyl choline	as labeled
Niacin	500–2,000 mg
Octacosanol	as labeled
L-tyrosine	1,000–2,000 mg
L-glutamine	500 mg
Boron	1–2 mg
Vitamin E	400–600 IU
Pycnogenol	50–150 mg

8

Preventing Cataracts

A cataract is a clouding of the eye lens. Cataracts can progress from where the vision is merely fogged or has "stars" to complete blindness. It used to be thought that cataracts came with age. Now it is known that cataracts are the result of long exposure to ultraviolet energy from the sun.

The ultraviolet "rays" are not visible; thus it is incorrect to call ultraviolet energy ultraviolet "light." However, common usage refers to this energy as ultraviolet light, and I will do so occasionally here for simplicity. The good news is that cataracts are not only entirely preventable—they are also reversible!

About twenty million people in the world are blinded by cataracts, and more than a million a year have operations to remove them in the United States.

Visible light passes through the eye lens and does no damage. Ultraviolet "B" energy is absorbed by compounds in the lens and releases free radicals.[1] Free radicals damage the normally clear proteins in the eye lens, forming cross-linked proteins and by-products that cloud the lens. Antioxidant nutrients can scavenge the free radicals and neutralize them before they can do damage to the eye lens. The wearing of hats and ultraviolet-absorbing sunglasses also helps by reducing the amount of ultraviolet light that impacts on the eye lens.

A study of Chesapeake Bay watermen by the Wilmer Eye Institute at Johns Hopkins University showed that heavy doses of sunlight make a person three times as likely to develop cataracts.[2] The study also found that wearing a hat with a wide brim reduced the ultraviolet light reaching the eye by 50%. Sunglasses can block the harmful ultraviolet rays by 60% to 95%.

In India, Dr. K. Seetharam Bhat measured the copper and zinc levels in healthy eyes and eyes having cataracts. The eyes with cataracts were lower in copper and zinc. These two minerals are incorporated into the superoxide dismutase (SOD) molecule. SOD is the main antioxidant in the eye lens that protects the lens against oxidative damage.

The level of vitamin E in the eye, especially the retina, decreases with age, according to epidemiological studies. These data do not necessarily apply to the individual, but this is a common observation among members of various age groups.

Protective Nutrients

Supplements that protect against cataracts include vitamins B-2, C, and E; beta-carotene; folic acid; the minerals selenium, copper, and zinc; the bioflavonoid quercetin; and, to a very limited extent, SOD. Normal ranges of supplementation will be adequate for this protection.

Researchers at the University of Western Ontario in London, Ontario confirmed an earlier U.S. study showing that vitamin C prevents cataracts, and they found that vitamin E did, too.[3-8] The researchers had previously shown that diabetic mice that were prone to cataracts were protected by vitamin E.

In studies by Drs. J. R. Trevithick, James McD. Robertson, and Allan Donner it was found that persons taking at least 400 IU of vitamin E and 300 milligrams of vitamin C supplements daily were largely *free of cataracts*. People who took only vitamin E supplements had 56% fewer cataracts, and those taking only vitamin C showed a 70% reduction. This once again verifies the synergism of the two antioxidant nutrients. I believe that when selenium is also included in the study, the synergistic effect will be tremendous.

Dr. P. Jacques and colleagues at Tufts University found that vitamin C and folic acid help prevent cataracts.[9] Their results showed those persons with the highest dietary intakes of vitamin C and folic acid were least likely to develop cataracts.

The Tufts University researchers led by Dr. P. Jacques also found a correlation between high blood levels of vitamins C, and E or beta-carotene and a low incidence of cataracts.[10] They concluded, "Our results suggest that individuals with high plasma levels of two or more of those vitamins thought to influence antioxidant status appear to have a reduced risk of cataract." Come on, gang, let's be conservative!

Nutrition Reviews discussed the relation of antioxidant vitamins in 1989.[11]

Supplement Program to Prevent Cataracts

If you are exposed to sunlight often or have cataracts forming, you may wish to consider the following supplements. I have had many people tell me that antioxidants have even reduced their existing cataracts.

TABLE 8.1
Supplements for Cataract Prevention

Nutrient	Range
Vitamin E	200–600 IU
Vitamin C	500–2,000 mg
Vitamin B-2	15–75 mg
Beta-carotene	5,000–15,000 IU
Folic acid	400–800 mcg
Selenium	100–200 mcg
Copper	1–3 mg
Zinc	10–20 mg
Quercetin	100–500 mg
Pycnogenol	50–150 mg

9

Easing Menopause

Menopause is not a disease, but it can seem like much more than a "change of life," according to about 25% of the women going through it. Medical authorities are still describing the conventional drug treatment with hormones as risky, but the evidence is debatable. If you believe that the drugs are indeed risky, then you may be pleased to know that safe nutrients can also relieve the problems of menopause.

In 1974 I conducted a survey of vitamin E users to learn why people took the supplement and whether it helped them. To my surprise, the survey resulted in my also receiving letters from thousands of women describing the unkind problems of menopause and how vitamin E helped them.

My research had been confined primarily to studying aging and cancer in laboratory animals, but since I had found vitamin E to help slow aging and prevent cancer, people kept asking me if vitamin E helped fight heart disease, too. The scientific and medical literature did not contain much in the way of well-designed clinical studies, so I had to start at the beginning.

The survey questionnaire did not mention menopause. I knew of no connection between vitamin E and menopause at the time. My laboratory mice had never mentioned it. But

when the readers of *Prevention* magazine returned the vitamin E survey questionnaire to me, I learned a lot. In the
following decade I learned a lot more about other nutrients
and their effect on menopause.

The most frequent comment was "vitamin E gave me relief
of hot flashes and other problems of menopause." Other
comments also caught me by surprise. I am not a social
historian, but I thought that women were liberated before
1974. Maybe the movement hadn't made its way through the
entire medical profession at that time.

The letters implied that physicians used to ignore the subject or treat it very superficially. One lady who had been in
nursing school during the 1940s reported that male physicians told her that menopause was all in the woman's head—
that it didn't exist. Other women told me that they suffered as
silently as possible because of the lack of understanding of
their husbands and the disinterest of their doctors.

By the 1960s physicians were freely prescribing tranquilizers, and by the 1970s hormones were widely prescribed. Both medications can present problems for some
women, while vitamin E can work as well—or better in some
cases.

Hormone replacement therapy can help some women keep
youthful skin and a healthy sex life. In European studies, this
long-term use of hormones has been shown to increase the
risk of breast cancer by 10%.[1] However, short-term use just
to relieve symptoms during menopause was not found to
increase the risk of breast cancer.

There are still questions raised about estrogens and endo-
metrial cancer and cervical cancer; this is a matter to discuss
with your gynecologist. However, if you choose not to take
such medicines, or if you still need additional help, vitamin
E, the minerals magnesium and calcium, and the amino acids
L-tryptophan and L-tyrosine will win a special place in your
heart.

Normally, menopause is a process in which the ovaries
gradually reduce their production of estrogen, a female sex
hormone, over a period of several years. Typically, menopause affects women between thirty-eight and fifty-five years
of age. A notable exception to this is the surgical menopause
caused by hysterectomy.

As the ovaries decrease their estrogen production the

body's hormonal balance is disturbed. After five or more years of this decline the ovaries essentially cease estrogen production, but the adrenal glands continue to make some estrogen. Eventually the body adjusts to the lower level of estrogen, and a new hormonal balance is established. However, during the adjustment period there can be great upheaval in the hypothalamus, which is the hormone control center. The hypothalamus occasionally becomes erratic, which is the cause of hot flashes, irritability, depression, anxiety, hyperactivity, tremors, fatigue, insomnia, dizziness, weight gain, sweats, vaginal dryness, and other problems. Wow, what a jolt to the system!

Well, since the hypothalamus is in the head, perhaps the doctors who used to say menopause was "all in a woman's head" were partially right.

Although the symptoms of menopause are extremely upsetting and uncomfortable, there are more serious long-term problems due to decreased estrogen production. One problem is stickier blood cells—increased blood-platelet adhesion. Sticky blood cells can clot and cause a heart attack. Another problem is osteoporosis, the thinning and weakening of bones. This will be discussed in the following chapter.

Fortunately, the nutrients that help ease menopause also protect against sticky blood and osteoporosis. The role of vitamin E in blood-platelet adhesion will be discussed in Chapter 19, and the role of calcium in bone health is discussed in the next chapter. Right now, let's discuss their role in easing menopause.

The older medical literature contains many studies showing the benefits of vitamin E in menopause. However, with the advent of tranquilizers and replacement hormones, nutritional approaches were discarded. Drug salesmen known as "detail men" call upon doctors to inform them of the wonders of their products, but there are no salesmen calling upon physicians to sell them on the virtues of vitamins. Vitamins are not patented and are inexpensive. Thus, there is not enough of a profit margin or monopoly to warrant salesmen to call on doctors.

In 1945 Dr. C. J. Christy reported in the *American Journal of Gynecology* that "the entire group of cases responded to the vitamin E treatment and showed either complete relief or very marked improvement. No untoward after-effects were noted. In some cases, relief of vasomotor instability was more easily obtained with vitamin E than with the use of estrogen; however, the chief advantage of vitamin E over estrogens is its freedom of stimulative effect on the genital system or on the parenchyma of the breast. Because vitamin E has no carcinogenic (cancer-causing) effect, it may be used quite freely in menopausal patients suffering from neoplasm."

Dr. H. Ferguson reported in the *Virginia Medical Monthly* in 1948 that "sixty of sixty-six patients with severe menopausal symptoms were completely relieved with 15 to 30 IU of vitamin E daily." In my survey, I found that most women obtained excellent results at 400 to 600 IU of vitamin E daily. I can't help but wonder—if the other six women had taken more vitamin E, would they have been helped too?

In a report on my survey findings that I published in *Prevention* magazine I described several other clinical studies.[2] Here are some brief excerpts from the medical reports: "Vitamin E therapy administered for long periods in doses of about 300 IU definitely benefitted patients with disagreeable menopausal symptoms. . . ." "After two years with trials in comparison with estrogen therapy, vitamin E has been found to be effective and free from undesirable side effects. . . ." "Treatment of patients with menopausal symptoms with vitamin E showed splendid results in practically all cases. It is recommended as preferable to estrogenic treatment. . . ." "Vitamin E was found to have a definite normalizing effect on menstrual functions and on menopausal phenomena. Vitamin E prevented the objectional symptoms of pain, irregularity, irritability, etc. which had been previously associated with the menstrual periods of these women. Women with the disagreeable symptoms associated with the change of life were relieved by vitamin E."

The medical reports continue into the 1950s and early 1960s. Dr. Evan Shute made several clinical studies in the 1950s that led to the famous books by his brother Wilfrid and himself.[3,4]

Here are examples of the survey findings from *Prevention* readers. "Vitamin E stopped my hot flashes." "Vitamin E prevented a hysterectomy in 1958." "Vitamin E eliminated the need for estrogen shots."

"Corrected vaginal dryness. It's *great—GREAT !!!*" "Vitamin E took care of the hot flashes and night sweats completely. I ran out of vitamin E for two months and started having heavy night sweats again. I started back again with vitamin E and have had no symptoms since. I will never be without vitamin E again."

Supplements

Well, so much for the benefits. Let's look at the supplements and intake ranges often used for relief of menopausal symptoms.

TABLE 9.1
Nutrients for Menopause

Nutrient	Range
Vitamin E	400–800 IU
Calcium	250–600 mg
Magnesium	300–600 mg
L-tryptophan (for nerves)	250–500 mg
L-tyrosine (for depression)	250–500 mg

10

Osteoporosis

Osteoporosis is a bone disease that causes brittle bones and/or a hump in the back. Often when you hear that an elderly person has fallen and broken a hip, it really was the opposite—the person's hip fractured due to the brittle bone, and then the person fell. Osteoporosis accounts for some eight million spontaneous bone fractures that occur in women every year.

The hump in the back is caused by the shrinkage or collapse of portions of the vertebrae. Ninety percent of postmenopausal women lose a significant amount of bone tissue, and twenty-six percent of women over the age of sixty years have loss of height involving pain and deformity. Four times as many women as men get osteoporosis, but estrogen loss doesn't explain osteoporosis in men.

In women, osteoporosis begins prior to menopause, but the rate of calcium loss from bones accelerates after menopause. Osteoporosis is not a free-radical disease. Osteoporosis is the result of poor diet, inadequate exercise, and genetics. Most people think in terms of the mineral calcium concerning bone health, but there are more nutrients involved.

Calcium forms the major structural compounds, but several other nutrients are involved in the "cement" that holds healthy bone together. Other major nutrients include silicon, vitamin D, vitamin K, phosphorus, zinc, manganese, boron, molybdenum, copper, strontium, and magnesium. Fluoride does not seem to be beneficial in spite of several poorly designed studies that originally held some promise. Later, better-designed tests showed the bone changes induced by fluoride did not reduce fractures or prevent osteoporosis.[1]

Osteoporosis involves decreased bone mass, including both minerals and proteins. The chemical composition of the remaining bone is unchanged. (In osteomalacia only the mineral content is lowered.)

The body contains more calcium than any other mineral, and 99% of it is in the bones and teeth. Many people are surprised to learn that the calcium within teeth and bone is not a permanent part of the structure. Bone calcium is continually being deposited and resorbed. It is in a constant state of flux. In fact, the form of bone calcium may change as we age.

Bone consists of calcium phosphate deposited within a soft, fibrous matrix. Calcium phosphate is a compound that is made from the minerals calcium and phosphorus, plus oxygen. However, this compound can exist in several physical forms. Calcium phosphate can be deposited in skeletal tissue to be highly crystalline and complexed with calcium hydroxide (a compound of calcium, hydrogen, and oxygen) to form a composition similar to the mineral ore hydroxyapatite, or the calcium phosphate can be non-crystalline.

Calcium is constantly being exchanged between bone and blood. This exchange is more rapid during the early years than the later years. In an adult male, it is estimated that about 700 milligrams of calcium enter and leave the bones each day.

The mineral content of bone is about 65% of its dry weight, with the bone protein matrix (mostly collagen) being the remaining 35%. "Fresh" bone contains about 20% moisture. Besides calcium (24%) and phosphorus (10%), the other minerals with known biological function include sodium, magnesium, manganese, chlorine, molybdenum, boron, silicon, and zinc. Molybdenum and zinc are involved in enzymes that help build bone. Other minerals are present, but whether or not they have function or merely accumulate is not agreed upon. I have listed those nutrients that my experience has taught me are important in the supplement section.

The incidence of osteoporosis (literally "hole-y bones") is greater among persons having low dietary calcium intake.[2] In osteoporosis, bone calcium is "borrowed" from the bone to maintain the critical blood level of calcium. This blood calcium level is so critical that it is under hormonal control. Calcium is also continually excreted from the body and consumed in other functions. As calcium reserves dwindle calcium excretion is lessened as more is reabsorbed, and calcium absorption from the intestine becomes more efficient, but there is still a net loss.

A major study shows that getting a moderate increase above the 1980 RDA for calcium, 800 milligrams per day, protected against hip fractures.[3] Thus, when the 1989 RDAs were published, it was not surprising to find a new calcium RDA of 1,000 milligrams per day. Government surveys have also shown that more than 60% of women were not getting even the lower former RDA of 800 milligrams.[4] The median U.S. intake of calcium is 450 to 500 milligrams per day.

A 1990 study showed that supplementing the diet with extra calcium significantly increased bone density.[5] Several other studies confirm the relationship.[6-14]

In 1984 Dr. Michael Horowitz and his colleagues at the Royal Adelaide Hospital in Australia published the results of their study in the *American Journal of Clinical Nutrition*. The researchers concluded that therapy with calcium supplements, which have no serious side effects, decreases bone resorption in postmenopausal osteoporosis. They noted that previous studies have shown that supplements of one to two and a half grams of calcium per day reduced the incidence of vertebral fracture by 50% and that supplements of one gram of calcium daily protected healthy postmenopausal women against osteoporosis.

Boron

We have now learned that boron is involved in protecting women against osteoporosis. Boron does not appear to be part of the bone matrix, but it is involved in building bone. Boron markedly exerts a positive effect on the male sex hormone testosterone and the female sex hormone estradiol. Boron also increases vitamin D formation; improves calcium, magnesium, potassium, and phosphorus retention; and is involved with methionine metabolism.

It appears that boron may be needed to activate (hydroxylate) specific steroid hormones such as vitamin D, testosterone, and estradiol.

A 1986 study by Drs. Forrest Nielsen and Curtiss Hunt determined that boron is significant in determining the incidence of osteoporosis.[15] In the study, boron supplements of three milligrams per day markedly improved several measures of bone health, such as reducing the excretion of calcium, phosphorus, and magnesium. Within eight days of boron supplementation the subjects lost 40% less calcium, 33% less magnesium, and slightly less phosphorus in their urine. At the same time, estradiol levels were increased.

Later, this same research team found that low-boron diets decreased blood levels of the active form of calcium and raised levels of calcitonin, a calcium-reducing hormone.[16]

Silicon

Silicon is a mineral that builds stronger bones and arteries. It may be involved in compounds similar to mucopolysaccharides (glycosaminoglycans) to form a "gluelike" substance in the bone matrix. Silicon is concentrated in sites of active calcification in bones.[17] Silicon deficiency results in abnormal bone formation.

Phosphates

Several studies show that the excessive phosphates in many women's diets weaken bones and encourage osteoporosis. Phosphates are compounds that include the mineral phosphorus, oxygen, and other elements. Dr. Isaac Schiff of Harvard Medical School confirms that women who drink soda regularly are more likely to suffer broken bones after age forty. Drinking an average of a can and a half daily doubles the risk of bone fractures in women over forty years of age.[18] Women tend to consume more diet cola, thinking it is a low-calorie drink that does little harm. Cola is high in phosphorus.

High blood phosphate levels increase the output of para-hormone, which stimulates the decalcification of bones. Phosphates also bind with magnesium and reduce body magnesium levels.

Supplements

A good diet plus exercise is important for good bone health and the prevention of osteoporosis. With so many women cutting back on calories to maintain a "chic" appearance, mineral supplements are a necessity.

The National Institutes of Health Consensus Conference on Osteoporosis in 1984 and the American Society for Bone and Mineral Research in 1982 both recommended that dietary calcium intake should be 1,000 milligrams per day for premenopausal women and 1,500 milligrams for postmenopausal women. In 1987 the experts met again at NIH and concluded that all Americans should get at least 1,000 milligrams of calcium daily. Thus, it was not unexpected to see a higher RDA published in 1989.

There is adequate phosphorus in most diets, especially from sodas and additives. Busy women may wish to consider their possible needs for the supplements in Table 10.1.

TABLE 10.1
Supplements for Bone Health

Nutrient	Daily Amount
Calcium	400–800 mg
Boron	2–3 mg
Silicon	15–25 mg
Copper	1–2 mg
Magnesium	300–500 mg
Manganese	5–10 mg
Zinc	10–20 mg
Molybdenum	100–200 mcg

11

Prostate and Impotence

The problems most feared by men, after heart disease, are becoming impotent and developing prostate trouble. Both, in spite of howls of protest from uninformed skeptics, have a large nutritional component. One factor, prostaglandins, is discussed in several chapters—please check the index and review those sections if you are not familiar with them. To say that prostaglandins have something to do with the prostate is an understatement. Prostaglandins were so named because the first prostaglandin studied originated in the prostate gland.

All of the nutrients involved in the production of prostaglandins, especially the polyunsaturated fatty acid precursors and the mineral zinc, are important factors in the health of the prostate. But let's start our discussion of the prostate by examining common prostate problems.

The healthy prostate gland weighs about an ounce and has a size somewhere between that of a large olive and that of a small walnut. The prostate gland consists of three globes that surround the urethra near the base of the penis. The urethra is the tube that carries urine from the bladder to the outside. The only known function of the prostate is to make the seminal fluid for ejaculation and to add it to the semen in the prostatic urethra.

The prostate gland can enlarge to the size of a plum or even a grapefruit. Enlarged prostate glands affect 10% of forty-year-old and 80% of eighty-year-old men. However, they are rare among men who are well nourished with zinc and omega-3 fatty acids such as eicosapentaenoic acid to make the prostaglandins. As a result, the healthy prostate stores a lot of zinc and omega-3 fatty acids. The testes also store a lot of zinc, which is needed to make semen.

There are three common prostate disorders. Prostatitis is an inflammation of the prostate gland that affects primarily younger men. Benign prostatic hypertrophy is an enlarged prostate gland that affects primarily older men. The swollen prostate tends to prevent the bladder from being completely emptied, thus resulting in a need for frequent urination. The third common disease of the prostate is cancer. This cancer normally affects older men and is often difficult to detect in its early stages.

Prostate cancer seems to have a free-radical link, which will be discussed later in Chapter 12. However, it also seems to have some link to sunshine. Sunshine, hence vitamin D, seems to be protective, as can be readily seen by looking at a map of prostate cancer incidence by county. It's almost as if the U.S. is divided in half, with those below the midline having much less prostate cancer—it's warmer, so the skin is exposed more to sunlight.

All three prostate diseases can have serious consequences. Your doctor should be consulted whenever symptoms appear. Do not wait to see if the symptoms go away or decide to try the "alternative" nutritional adjunct first. You can start the "prudent" measures while you also start the "alternative" measures as an adjunct. Prostate troubles are signaled by pain or difficulty in urination or sex.

Zinc

Popular nutritional therapies for prostate troubles include zinc supplements or pumpkin seeds, which are good sources of zinc and polyunsaturated fatty acids. Such "therapies" are popular for one reason—they work!

Unfortunately, most diets are slightly deficient in zinc, and as we age we tend to use more zinc (for example, to make semen and insulin) than we take in. As a result, the prostate struggles to produce prostaglandins, and the gland compensates by enlarging itself.

Several studies have shown that this enlargement could be reduced by adequate intake of zinc in about 85% of men. However, some men don't respond to zinc therapy because they also have an omega-3 deficiency.

In another clinical trial of zinc, poor results were obtained because the zinc supplement was poorly absorbed. It is not a question of how much zinc you eat, but how much zinc becomes available to the prostate. We have now discovered the form of zinc that is best utilized by the prostate. This form is zinc picolinate.

Many people have reported success with sunflower and pumpkin seeds, and even oysters. The sunflower and pumpkin seeds are rich sources of zinc and omega-3 fatty acids. Oysters are a rich source of zinc, and I am willing to speculate that they are also a good source of omega-3 fatty acids, but I haven't gotten that far yet with my research.

That zinc is effective is not really surprising when you consider all of the relationships between zinc and male sexual development and function. Zinc deficiency in childhood leads to impaired development of the male sex organs and secondary sexual characteristics. In adulthood, zinc is vital to the testes and testosterone production. Even a marginal zinc deficiency can lower one's libido.

Diets even moderately low in zinc produce reduced sperm counts. Zinc deficiency can produce sterility. In such cases, supplemental zinc returns the sperm count to normal in a few months.

In a study at various Chicago hospitals of two hundred men having prostatitis not caused by bacterial infection, zinc supplements relieved the symptoms in 70% of the men, and their prostates returned to normal or near-normal size.[1]

There is no reason for the prostate to enlarge due to age. A clinical trial involving nineteen men having benign prostatic hypertrophy found that zinc supplements brought relief to all nineteen patients, but more importantly, the prostate returned to normal size in fourteen of the nineteen men.[2]

Palm Berries

Recently there has been considerable interest in palm berries (saw palmetto fruit—*Serenoa repens* or *Sabal serrulata*). They are rich in fatty acids and zinc, but the important factor is that they are rich in biologically active sterols and beta-sitosterols.

It has been postulated that the buildup of testosterone in the prostate encourages the conversion of testosterone to dihydrotestosterone (DHT). The DHT stimulates the prostate cells to proliferate so as to enlarge the gland. It is believed that the saw palmetto sterols block the conversion of testosterone into DHT and prevent the gland's enlargement.

In a clinical trial involving 110 men, 50 were given 160 milligrams of saw palmetto fruit extract twice a day. Of these, 14 were greatly improved and 31 were moderately improved. Only five did not improve. The number of midnight visits to the bathroom was cut in half, and the urine output increased by 50%.[3]

Another plant extract that is showing promise is pygeum (*Pygeum africanum* or *Prunnus africana*). Extracts from the pygeum contain sterols, pentacylic triterpenoids, and ferulic esters. Keep an eye out for studies that might show if it is safe and efficacious.

Supplements for Prostate Problems

You and your health professional may wish to consider the dietary supplement ranges listed in Table 11.1 as an adjunct to conventional prostate gland treatments.

IMPOTENCE

Much has been written about impotence, but only recently have scientists uncovered the biochemistry that links many

TABLE 11.1
Nutrients for Prostate Protection

Nutrient	Daily Amount
Zinc	75–150 mg (reduce to 25–50 mg after two weeks)
Eicosapentaenoic acid (EPA)	4–8 capsules
or	
Evening primrose oil (GLA)	4–8 capsules
Selenium	50–200 mcg
Magnesium	200–400 mg
Vitamin B-6	25–50 mg
Vitamin D	300–600 IU
Vitamin E	100–400 IU
Vitamin C	250–500 mg
Pumpkin seeds	as desired
or	
Saw palmetto fruit extract	320 milligrams
or	
Saw palmetto berries	1 oz.

organic forms of impotence. This biochemical pathway seems to have a dietary component. This is not to claim that there are food supplements to cure impotence, but a suggestion that diet can affect impotence. Surely diabetes and atherosclerosis affect the flow of blood to the penile arteries that permit erection. But there is a suggestion that diet may play an additional role. This is not a discussion of psychological impotence or aphrodisiacs.

Much of our recent knowledge concerning the biochemistry of impotence has come from a research team headed by Dr. Arnold Melman of the Veterans Administration Center at the Indiana University Medical Center in Indianapolis. Dr. Melman and his colleagues found that the common link between the various causes of organic erectile impotence was a decrease in the content of the neurotransmitter norepinephrine. This finding seems to be true for various causes, including diabetes mellitus, neurologic disorders, intrinsic disease of the penis, and treatment with various drugs for high blood pressure or beta-blockers for heart disease.

Studies have shown that penile erection is achieved via postganglionic sympathetic adrenergic innervation in concert with parasympathetic neurons. A deficiency in the nerve chemical messenger would prevent erection. Animal experiments confirmed that agents that would block or deplete the neurotransmitter did indeed cause impotence.

Studies have also shown that the nerve is intact, but lacking a supply of the neurotransmitter.[4-7] If this is the case, then it is very likely—but to my knowledge untested—that the dietary amino acid L-tyrosine can circulate in the bloodstream to nourish the penile neurons so as to normalize norepinephrine production and restore penile erectile function. It is certainly worth a try and is a sensible alternative to the alternative.

French scientists studying the chemistry of arousal note that since the normal progression of the process depends on the ability of the mast cells of the genitals to produce histamine as required, folic acid is important. Also, heavy excesses of niacin, such as one might use to lower cholesterol, should be reduced if impotence is a problem. No, I didn't say that niacin excess caused impotence. I said that when impotence already exists due to other causes, heavy excesses of niacin may interfere with the histamine buildup.

Herbs

In addition to the nutrients discussed above, several herbs have shown good potential for curing certain types of impotence. A study reported in the *Journal of Urology* showed that the herb ginkgo biloba was effective in impotency caused by reduced penile blood flow. Sixty patients who did not respond to other treatments were given 60 milligrams of ginkgo biloba daily. Noticeable improvements in penile blood flow were measured in six to eight weeks in many patients, with half *regaining full potency within six months*.

Another herb has shown promise at Stanford University and in Canadian research,[8-10] but we should wait for more safety and efficacy studies before drawing any conclusions. This herb is yohimbe *(Pausinystalia johimbe)*, and its active compound is yohimbine. Yohimbine dilates surface blood vessels and encourages the release of norepinephrine.

Supplements That May Help Alleviate Impotence

As you are working with your health professional you may wish to consider the following as an adjunct therapy:

TABLE 11.2
Nutrients to Alleviate Impotence

Nutrient	Daily Amount
L-tyrosine	1,000–3,000 mg
Vitamin B-6	25–50 mg
Vitamin E	100–400 IU
Zinc	50–150 mg
Folic Acid	400–800 mcg
Magnesium	200–400 mg
(Yohimbe)	see your doctor
(Ginkgo)	see your doctor

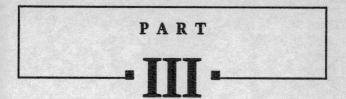

PART

▪ III ▪

Supernutrition
Against Cancer

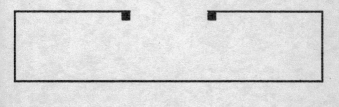

12

Preventing Cancer

———————————————————■———————————————————

Other scientists examining my early research on slowing the aging process suggested that I may not really be altering the "primary aging process" but instead may be lengthening life span by preventing diseases such as cancer. I felt that free radicals were involved in the primary aging process, but I still checked out the suggestion from my colleagues. After all, both aging and disease prevention could be involved.

My data did show the cancer incidence in my laboratory animals was less than half of the normal rate. I expanded my research to cancer prevention and found the antioxidant nutrients were synergistic in cancer prevention.

When cancer-causing chemicals were put in the mouse diets, those receiving standard amounts of nutrients developed cancer at the expected high rates. However, those animals protected with extra antioxidant nutrients developed only a fraction of the expected cancers.

My experiments were conducted with several antioxidants selected so that their synergism would provide protection at low concentrations. The incidence of stomach cancer to be expected in mice fed sufficient amounts of a chemical called dimethylbenzantracene (DMBA) is 85% to 90%. That rate can be reduced to between 5% and 15% with antioxidant nutrients.

When I used strains of laboratory mice that inherently had high cancer rates without having to add cancer-causing chemicals to their diets, the results were the same.

When only one antioxidant nutrient was used at high levels, sometimes the induced cancer would not show up where expected but would be found in another organ. The combination of antioxidants totally prevented the induced cancers.[1,2]

Antioxidant nutrients not only provide a first line of defense by destroying free radicals before they damage the body, they also provide three other lines of defense. The second defense is maintaining liver health. The healthy liver can detoxify many carcinogens.

A third line of defense is the barrier of each cell—the cell membrane. Antioxidants protect cell membranes so that carcinogens can't enter the cells and cells don't reproduce wildly due to their membrane-sensing mechanism being damaged.

The Immune System, Cancer, and AIDS

The last line of defense is the immune system. Even if a precancerous cell is formed, a healthy immune system will identify this abnormal cell and destroy it. An immune system impaired by poor nutrition will be unable to perform either function.

Antioxidants also enhance the immune system. Vitamin E enhances the immune system by regulating prostaglandins.[3] Vitamin C and dimethylglycine are also immune enhancers. In addition, vitamin C is also an in vitro antiviral. Recent studies have shown vitamin C inactivates human immunodeficiency virus replication [Harakeh, Steve, et al. Proc. Natl. Acad. Sci. 87:7245–9 (Sep. 1990)].

To understand the many factors that control the health of the immune system, one should have an understanding of this amazing system (see page 90 for a simplified but thorough description).

Clinical Trials Are Under Way

Okay, mice and rats may not develop cancer exactly the same way we do. However, rodents are the standard research tool that has taught us most of what we know about cancer at this writing. Rodents may be more susceptible to mutations and oxidative damage than people. So we can't base our preventive actions solely on the results of laboratory-animal experiments.

After thoroughly testing my premise in other laboratories, scientists began looking at real people in what are called epidemiological studies. In essence, they examined what people ate and their cancer incidence. Many studies confirmed that *people* who ate more of the antioxidant nutrients had lower rates of cancer.

This "looking back" type of study with statistics doesn't really prove that the antioxidant nutrients prevent cancer either. But the studies do lend considerable support to the hypothesis that this is indeed the case. Conclusive proof lies in "forward-looking" clinical trials. These trials are being conducted by the U.S. government.

While the clinical trials are being conducted—which will take several years—the U.S. government and the American Cancer Society are recommending diets rich in antioxidant nutrients. The National Cancer Institute is sponsoring several prospective clinical trials as a final test of antioxidant nutrients' cancer protection. There were at least a dozen long-term, large-scale clinical trials involving selenium and fourteen involving beta-carotene under way in 1990. These studies, involving the prevention of cancers of the lung, breast, colon, skin, stomach, and esophagus, are being conducted around the world: in the United States, in Europe, in China, and in Africa.

At a scientific conference in Boca Raton during the spring of 1987, Dr. Peter Greenwald, director of the Division of Cancer Prevention and Control for the National Cancer Institute, pointed out, "There is now general scientific consensus that about 80% of cancer cases appear to be linked to the way people live their lives. For example, whether or not we

THE IMMUNE SYSTEM

The body protects itself against invasion by disease microorganisms through its ability to recognize itself and to reject and destroy everything that is nonself. The mechanism that accomplishes this is the immune system.

The immune system is a complex network of lymphocytes (white blood cells formed in the lymph tissue), macrophages (large scavenger white blood cells), antibodies (proteins that can react with specific germs), and interferon (an antiviral, antitumor compound).

The immune system produces three types of lymphocytes, called T-cells, B-cells, and K-cells. The T-cells have the ability to reject all foreign matter, while the B-cells have the ability to produce antibodies. Relatively little is understood about the T-cells and the B-cells, but even less is known about the "killer" K-cells, which are involved in an immune phenomenon called "antibody-dependent cell-mediated cytotoxicity."

All three lymphocytes are formed from the same basic cell of the bone marrow, called a "stem cell." Stem cells are transformed into T-cells in the thymus, and B-cells may be produced in the bone marrow.

These specialized lymphocyte cells (B-, T-, and K-cells) are stored in the lymphoid tissues such as the lymph nodes in the armpits, behind the ears, in the groin, and in other locations.

When an invader (antigen) is detected the immune system responds by releasing one or more of its specialized lymphocytes. Released T-cells multiply and surround the invader. Once the invader has been isolated by rings of T-cells, it is chemically attacked by these defenders. The T-cells can also summon macrophages from the reticuloendothelial system to digest the invader.

The B-cells can also be released; they then produce antibodies (immunoglobulins) that stick to the invader, thereby increasing the likelihood of its ingestion by macrophages. Antibodies immunoglobulin M (I_gM) and immunoglobulin G (I_gG) circulate in the blood, while immunoglobulin A (I_gA) circulates in the saliva and fluids that bathe the mucous membranes. At least one other antibody, immunoglobulin E (I,E) exists, but little is known about it.

Antibodies are tailor-made to specifically lock onto each of the millions of different microorganisms that may invade a person. Macrophages cleanse the blood and lymph of foreign particulate matter and also produce interferon, the body's antiviral compound.

---

smoke, the foods we eat, and certain industrial pollutants all affect our likelihood of getting cancer. The role of diet in the cause and prevention of cancer is particularly important."

Dr. Greenwald told the conference, "One area that shows great promise is called chemoprevention. We are studying whether natural agents in pill or capsule form can reduce the incidence of cancer. We have some twenty-eight ongoing different chemoprevention studies of human populations right now. Among the compounds being tested are vitamin A, beta-carotene, vitamin C, vitamin E, vitamin B-6, vitamin B-12, folic acid, and selenium."

The results from these studies should begin appearing in the mid- to late 1990s. While the scientific and medical communities continue their research in cancer prevention, you should consider carefully the recommendations of the major cancer-prevention authorities: Include more vitamins A, C, and E, beta-carotene, and the trace mineral selenium in your diets.

The guidelines also suggest including more of the crucifer vegetables (*Brassica* genus)—cabbage, broccoli, cauliflower, and brussels sprouts. In the raw vegetables there is an appreciable amount of indole glycosinates. These indole compounds may act as free-radical scavengers, or they may stimulate the production of detoxifying enzymes. Future research will clarify the mechanism, but diets rich in these raw vegetables are associated with reduced risk of several cancers. When cooked, these vegetables have less than half of the indoles.

Other compounds that have not yet been shown to be nutrients, and which are thus not yet available as food supplements, are glucarate (from cruciferous vegetables) and ellagic acid (in fruits, nuts, and berries).

The guidelines are given in "Diet, Nutrition and Cancer Prevention" by the U.S. Public Health Service,[4] "Diet, Nutrition and Cancer" by the National Academy of Sciences,[5] the

Journal of the National Cancer Institute,[6] *Science* magazine,[7] and the *New England Journal of Medicine*.[8] The American Cancer Society has disseminated this advice through its own publication, "Cancer News."[9] This, in turn, was further disseminated as an article in the February 1983 *Reader's Digest*.[10]

Interesting Human Studies

There are hundreds of animal studies that show the protective effect of antioxidants against cancer. There are dozens of human studies that show the same. However, there is no need to review hundreds of studies. Six studies should make the point.

(1) Considering selenium blood levels alone, those persons in the lowest fifth of all blood selenium levels have twice the incidence of cancer of those in the highest fifth (Willett, 1983).[11]

(2) Total cancer mortality is three times higher in persons having blood selenium levels below a certain value than the incidence of cancer in those above this value (Yu, 1985).[12]

(3) Considering selenium blood levels alone, those persons in the lowest tenth of all blood selenium levels have six times the incidence of cancer of those in the highest tenth (Clark, 1984).[13]

(4) Both selenium and vitamin E are needed to prevent cancer (Horvath, 1983).[14]

(5) When considering both selenium and vitamin E blood levels, those persons in the lowest third of blood vitamin E levels and also having a low blood selenium level had more than eleven times the incidence of cancer of those in the upper two thirds of blood vitamin E and selenium levels (Salonen, 1985).[15]

(6) Another researcher concludes that "selenium should be considered not only as a preventative, but also as a therapeutic agent in cancer treatment and may act additively or synergistically with drug and radiation treatments" (Milner, 1984).[16]

Each of these studies will be examined in detail shortly,

but the brief synopses should hold your attention for a while. Let's look at one of the six studies for a moment to make a point about synergism and new knowledge over my earlier results.

Selenium and Vitamin E Must Both Be Amply Present

As I have often mentioned, the advantage of the combination of antioxidant nutrients is synergism. I discovered that in my early laboratory animal experiments. However, the more sophisticated studies of Drs. Paula Horvath and Clement Ip of Roswell Park Memorial Institute in Buffalo uncovered the exact mechanism for this synergism.

Most scientific studies examine one variable at a time to isolate the effect of just that one variable. This reduces confusion from confounding factors. Yet the body is not a simple laboratory. It is a biologically complex mechanism that functions independently of science's effort to study it.

Most researchers study the effect of one nutrient at a time, but in so doing they can easily miss not only the synergistic effect of vitamin E and selenium if they are not aware of it, but even worse, they can overlook any effect of either. The effect may be blurred by lumping all vitamin E data together and all selenium data together. The discovery of antioxidant synergism may be my greatest contribution to nutrition.

Drs. Ip and Horvath have not missed this point. In 1983 they performed a sophisticated study that showed why vitamin E and selenium are synergistic in preventing cancer. Their evidence indicates that it is not only the antioxidant protection of vitamin E in the membranes or the antioxidant protection of selenium-containing glutathione peroxidase. They found the critical factor is the amount of microsomal peroxidase activity that is stimulated only by the presence of both vitamin E and selenium.

The message here is that scientists should not be studying the correlation between the blood levels of one nutrient alone and the incidence of cancer. Studying selenium alone, we do in fact find that there is a substantial reduction in cancer risk with the higher blood levels of selenium. But we find the same relationship with vitamin E and some types of cancer—the more vitamin E in the blood, the lower the incidence of cancer. As an example, consider the report by Dr. Wald in the *British Journal of Cancer* that showed that women in the lowest quintile (fifth) of vitamin E levels had 5.2 times the incidence of cancer of women in the highest. However, when a person's blood is rich in both vitamin E and selenium, the protection given that person is far more than that of adding the vitamin E protection and the selenium protection together.

If a person has a normal blood level of selenium but is very deficient in vitamin E, that person will not have a good defense against cancer. Conversely, if a person is a little low in selenium but well fortified with vitamin E, then that person may be more resistant to cancer.

Since the vitamin E blood level can affect the usefulness of selenium, researchers should be looking at the combined levels, not at just a simple selenium level. Once other researchers catch on to this we will see even more dramatic results. This becomes apparent in the Finnish study by Dr. Salonen.

Dr. Jukka Salonen and his colleagues at the University of Kuopio (Finland) have been studying over 12,000 Finns for several years. The study is known as the North Karelia Project. Four years after drawing blood samples from these 12,155 persons, 51 had died of cancer. They were matched by age, sex, and smoking habits with others, and their blood samples were analyzed and compared.

In this study many factors were examined, but most important, vitamin E and selenium levels of the blood were examined *in combination*. The relative risk of cancer death for the third of people with blood selenium levels below 47 micrograms per liter of blood compared to those with higher levels was 5.8 to 1. But of more importance is the finding that, for people with low selenium levels who also had vitamin E levels in the lowest of values, risk of death from cancer compared to persons with both selenium and vitamin E levels in the upper two thirds of values was *11.4 to 1*.

Now here are the details of the human studies showing benefit from just one nutrient alone. Keep in mind that before epidemiological studies were done I and others had done hundreds of laboratory-animal studies to verify this protective effect.

A study that got a lot of people interested in cancer prevention and nutrition was the 1983 Willett study. This study was conducted by a well-respected group of researchers, and the work was done at major centers of learning: Harvard, Johns Hopkins, Duke, the University of Texas, and other respected institutions.

The results were published in a major medical journal rather than in an obscure scientific periodical. Many physicians read of the importance of blood selenium levels and their relationship to cancer risk for the first time thanks to the Willett study.

In the Willett study, blood samples had been collected in 1973 from 4480 men from 14 regions of the United States. At the time of collection of the blood samples, none of the men had detectable signs of cancer. The blood samples were preserved and stored for later analysis.

During the next five years 111 cases of cancer were detected in the group. The researchers then retrieved the stored blood samples from these men, and from 210 other men who were selected because they matched the newly developed cancer patients in age, sex, race, and smoking history. The levels of several nutrients and other factors were compared for the men who developed cancer and those men who remained free of cancer.

One difference stood out as being highly significant: The risk of cancer for subjects in the lowest quintile (fifth) of blood selenium levels was twice that of subjects in the highest.

Another Finnish study confirmed that vitamin E protects against cancer. Dr. R. Peto and colleagues evaluated blood vitamin E levels and subsequent cancer incidence in 21,000 Finnish men from six geographic areas. Vitamin E levels were measured from stored blood samples from 453 subjects who developed cancer during the follow-up of six to ten years. These levels were compared to those of 841 other men who did not develop cancer but were of the same age, lifestyle, etc.

The results showed that men with higher vitamin E levels

had a lower cancer risk. Associations were strongest in non-smokers and in younger age groups. Adjusted relative risks in the two highest quintiles of blood vitamin E levels compared to all other quintiles were 70% for all cancers combined and 60% for cancers unrelated to smoking.[17]

A Chinese study examined the relationship between blood levels of selenium in 1458 healthy adults in 24 regions of China. The study was led by Dr. Shu-Yu Yu of the Cancer Institute of the Chinese Academy of Medical Sciences in Beijing.

The researchers found that there was a statistically significant inverse correlation between age-adjusted cancer death rates and the selenium levels in the blood of local residents. In the areas with high selenium levels there was significantly lower cancer mortality. Total cancer mortality was three times higher in areas where mean blood selenium level was greater than 8 micrograms per deciliter of blood than where it was 11 microliters per deciliter.

Dr. Larry C. Clark and colleagues at Cornell determined the blood selenium levels in 240 skin cancer patients and compared the results of those from 103 apparently healthy persons living in low-selenium areas. The mean blood selenium level for the skin cancer patients was significantly lower than that of the apparently healthy individuals. After adjusting for age, sun damage to the skin, blood beta-carotene and vitamin A levels, and other factors, the incidence of skin cancer in those persons in the lowest decile (tenth) of blood selenium was 5.8 times as great as those in the highest decile.

Dr. John A. Milner of the University of Illinois has been studying selenium and cancer prevention for more than a decade. Most of Dr. Milner's studies involve transplanting or injecting cancer cells into mice receiving different levels of dietary selenium. He has found that selenium inhibits the development of such cancer.

Dr. Milner's conclusion is that selenium should be considered not only as a preventive, but also as a therapeutic agent in cancer treatment.

That's the same opinion reached by Dr. Lillian Pothier of the Roswell Park Memorial Institute. She studied seventy cancer patients and confirmed that they all had lower-than-normal blood levels of selenium. She also noted that many cancer treatments can further reduce blood selenium levels, and that common side effects such as susceptibility to infection, weakness, and muscle pain are results of selenium deficiency. She urged that selenium supplements be considered for all cancer patients.[18]

Cancer Regression

A few studies are appearing that show that antioxidants can cause cancers to regress. Vitamin E and beta-carotene together have reduced epidermal tumors in hamsters.[19]

Another researcher, who is now deceased, found that when blood levels of both vitamin E and selenium reached normal values, tumors would regress. It was not just how much was in the diet, but how much eventually reached the blood. The researcher was Dr. Richard C. Donaldson, assistant chief of surgery at the St. Louis Veterans Administration Hospital.

This book does not address the subject of cancer cure, which is a medical problem, not a nutritional problem. Nutrition is an important adjunct to cancer treatment. However, nutritional approaches should not be used alone, and no cancer patient should go without the best of medical diagnoses and treatments. New therapies are appearing each month, and older methods are becoming more effective with newer treatment variations.

However, for the sake of encouraging other researchers, I will discuss some of Dr. Donaldson's findings. Dr. Donaldson presented these results to his peers at the annual meeting of Veterans Administration surgeons in 1980 and to the National Cancer Institute on May 9, 1983. However, I am not aware of anyone following up on them. The data reported here are from progress reports made by Dr. Donaldson to one of the supporters of his research, and I will be happy to send complete copies to any medical researcher who requests them. I cannot send them to the general public.

At the time of Dr. Donaldson's presentation to the National Cancer Institute he had 140 patients enrolled in his study. According to his reports, all patients who entered his study were certified as being terminally ill by two physicians after receiving the appropriate conventional treatment for their particular cancer. Some of the patients who entered the study program with only weeks to live were alive and well after four years, and with no signs or symptoms of cancer. Not all patients were cured, but all had reduction in tumor size and pain. It is unfortunate that they did not receive the selenium and vitamin E until they were pronounced incurable. This research may well change cancer therapy in the future if researchers continue where Dr. Donaldson left off.

It is important to realize that the dramatic improvements did not occur until sufficient selenium was ingested to bring the patient's blood selenium level up to normal. Sometimes this could be achieved in a few weeks with 200 to 600 micrograms of selenium per day, while other individuals required as much as 2,000 micrograms per day to normalize the blood selenium levels.

No signs of toxicity were observed in any patient—even in the autopsies of the thirty-seven patients who were helped but not cured by the antioxidant therapy.

As an example, of eight patients with inoperable lung cancer, four were alive and well one year later, *with no signs of cancer as shown by x-ray examination*. Normally, all eight would have been expected to have died within that time.

In a March 9, 1979 letter Dr. Donaldson first reported the difficulty in normalizing the blood selenium levels of his terminal cancer patients. "It has been a surprise to me that cancer patients receiving up to 200 micrograms of selenium (tablet form) daily for up to two years continued to show low selenium levels in the range of 0.12 to 0.19 micrograms per 100 milliliters of blood. I then increased the dose to 900 micrograms daily for four patients—a recurrent brain tumor, a widely metastatic cancer of the prostate, an advanced nonoperable adenocarcinoma of the lung, and a recurrent squamous cell carcinoma of the face. *After thirty days, all four showed evidence of improvement, with two becoming outpatients.*"

After thirty days the blood selenium level increased to an average of 0.4 micrograms per 100 milliliters of blood. *"Associated with this rise has been a partial reduction in the size of tumors."*

Dr. Donaldson's May 11, 1979 report noted, "We are now

able, with 100% regularity, to increase the blood levels (of selenium) by nearly several fold by giving 1,000 to 2,000 micrograms of selenium daily and then dropping back to a maintenance dose. In a patient with prostate cancer with widespread metastases, *coinciding with the increase in (blood) selenium above 0.3 micrograms per 100 milliliters was a dramatic drop in acid phosphatase from 600 units to 100 units, complete clearing of blood in urine and an increase in appetite. His pain has been relieved approximately 90%. Patient is now an outpatient.*

"In a patient with salivary gland cancer, the cancer remained static at the lower dosage of 200 micrograms per day. When the dose was increased so that the blood level reached 0.3 micrograms per 100 milliliters, "the cancer regressed steadily until examination revealed no gross evidence of cancer and a completely patent right nasal passage.

"A patient with postradiation recurrence of squamous cell cancer in the right supraclavicular area developed paralysis of the right vocal cord and inability to swallow without aspiration of food into the trachea before adjustment of the selenium dosage to 1800 micrograms for five days and then to 900 micrograms daily. *Two days later, examination revealed softening of the neck tissues, relief of cord paralysis, and no problem swallowing. The patient was discharged* and continued on chemotherapy and antioxidants.

"As is evident, we are presented with many unanswered questions. Apparently, occasional patients with relatively low levels of selenium (0.2) can be associated with dramatic tumor regressions. For other patients, the regression is not evident until levels reach 0.4 to 0.5, while still others may require levels in excess of 0.8."

On August 17, 1979 Dr. Donaldson reported a patient with carcinoma in the mouth who had elected to go with chemo-immunotherapy plus selenium yeast sixteen months earlier. His cancer had regressed approximately 75%. There was still no reason to operate, or to give radiation therapy. "I feel that we are pursuing a safe, rational therapy schedule because I evaluate and treat the patient once a week so that standard therapy can be resorted to at any time the cancer appears to be expanding. Standard treatment in the beginning would have been a combined resection of one half of the mandible (jaw) plus a neck dissection. Needless to say, this patient is quite happy to have avoided radical, deforming surgery to date.

"Another patient with clinical evidence of melanoma in the form of numerous intradermal metastases in the left arm near the site of the primary has shown complete regression of some of these lesions. He has been receiving chemoimmunotherapy and selenium for five months. He is a real-estate agent working full-time."

A week later Dr. Donaldson wrote to another researcher, "Our long-term (six months to one year) results are well ahead of historical controls. A controlled study is in order. I like the theory that selenium uptake by cancer cells might make them more sensitive to chemoimmunotherapy."

I hope that physicians reading these results will follow up on Dr. Donaldson's clinical observations. What a great opportunity to make a major contribution to humanity!

Animal studies confirm that antioxidant nutrients can act synergistically to *regress tumors*. In hamsters having cancers, oral vitamin E and beta-carotene supplements were synergistic in regressing tumors.[20]

Although my research was concerned with the prevention of cancer, I have since learned that there were reports that selenium helped treat cancer already buried in the medical literature. In 1956 four leukemia patients were given selenocystine with the result of a rapid decrease in total leukocyte count and reduction in spleen size.[21]

In 1975 Dr. K. McConnell noticed a link in survival time in 110 cancer patients and their blood selenium levels. The patients with the lowest blood selenium levels had the most tumors, the most far-reaching cancer spread, and the shortest survival times.[22]

Drs. Raymond Shamberger and Charles Willis of the Cleveland Clinic found healthy persons between the ages of 50 and 71 to average 21.7 micrograms of selenium per 100 milliliters of blood, whereas cancer patients in the same age group averaged only 16.2 micrograms of selenium per 100 milliliters of blood. The worst cases had the lowest selenium levels, 13.7, 13.9 and 14.3.

An eight-year Swedish study of 10,000 men age 46 to 48 found that blood selenium levels were significantly lower in cancer patients.[23]

Vitamin C

As mentioned earlier, vitamin C strengthens the immune system and has antiviral properties. The role of vitamin C in cancer prevention and treatment is extensive. The best discussion of this is presented in "Cancer and Vitamin C" by Drs. Ewan Cameron and Linus Pauling (Norton & Co., 1979).

Fish Oil

There are several dozen studies showing that one nutrient or another is protective against cancer. Space doesn't allow the coverage of all the studies. The new studies on fish oil (EPA) and evening primrose oil (GLA) are very interesting.

Research suggests that diets high in fish oils may help prevent and arrest growth of breast, colon, prostate, and pancreatic cancers. Dr. Rashida Karmali of Rutgers University and Memorial Sloan-Kettering Hospital has found that fish oil counteracts the action of vegetable oils that promote harmful cell changes.

In Dr. Karmali's studies, which were reported to the 1986 annual meeting of the American Dietetic Association in Las Vegas, rats given corn oil were compared to those given corn oil plus fish oil. Those given the fish oil had significantly fewer and smaller breast tumors. Dr. Karmali's colon and prostate experiments also indicate that fish oil is protective against those cancers.

In an earlier study, Dr. Karmali's group had shown that EPA inhibited the growth of transplanted tumors (mammary adenocarcinoma). Fish oil (MaxEPA) was given orally to laboratory rats for one week before and three weeks after they received the transplants of cancer tissue. The laboratory animals were maintained on standard laboratory diets, with the exception that different groups were given different amounts of EPA. After three weeks tumor growth was significantly less in the three MaxEPA groups than in the unsupplemented controls.

Levels of arachidonic acid (AA) were higher in tumors

from laboratory animals given MaxEPA, and levels of prostaglandin and thromboxane products of AA metabolism were reduced. Tumor microsomes from animals given MaxEPA had decreased ability to synthesize AA metabolites. The researchers concluded that inhibition of AA metabolism may be a mechanism by which the formation of mammary cancer is reduced.[24]

In a study at Cornell University, rats injected with a chemical known to cause pancreatic cancer had fewer and smaller tumors with fish oil than with corn oil.[25] Dr. T. P. O'Connor and his colleagues concluded that "this study provides evidence that fish oils, rich in omega-3 fatty acids, may have potential as inhibitory agents in cancer development."

In another Cornell experiment, mice injected with cancer-causing chemicals had only one third as many tumors develop when fish oil was 20% of calories as opposed to corn oil being 20% of calories.[26]

A clinical trial by Tufts University researchers involving nine volunteers found that EPA had an anti-inflammatory effect and inhibited a tumor-promoting factor called "tumor necrosis factor."[27] Other studies lend confirming data.[28-30]

Dimethylglycine (DMG)

One nutrient, dimethylglycine (DMG), an amino acid, has been found to stimulate both branches of the immune tree. It is more accurate to describe DMG as a nutrient metabolite or nonfuel nutrient. DMG is produced in the body and enters into the metabolic process. DMG is found in foods such as liver, seeds, and nuts. Dietary DMG has positive effects in many areas, including increased energy production due to enhanced oxygen utilization and ranging to stimulation of the immune system.

Early research on DMG's effect on the immune system was carried out by a group at the Medical University of South Carolina at Charleston headed by Dr. Charles D. Graber. Their study, published in the *Journal of Infectious Diseases*, showed that *DMG enhances both humoral and cell-mediated immune responses in humans.*[31] The double-blind study of twenty human volunteers showed a fourfold increase in antibody response.

This was the first study to confirm the benefits in humans of DMG found in earlier animal studies. Later, animal studies at Clemson University by Drs. Elizabeth A. Reap and John W. Lawson expanded our knowledge of the immune-enhancing properties of DMG, ranging from protection against the flu to protection from melanoma.[32] They confirmed that "DMG appears to be effective in enhancing both the humoral and cellular branches of the immune system."

They noted, "Our results also show that DMG given orally can potentiate the immune response in a whole animal." They reported potentiation of the immune response ranging between fourfold and tenfold.

This information should be of interest not only in preventing cancer, but in protecting against many, many diseases, including AIDS. The scientists remarked, "in this report we show DMG's ability to enhance normal immune function. In addition, DMG might be helpful in diseases where immunologic integrity has been compromised. In immunosuppressive diseases such as acquired immunodeficiency syndrome (AIDS), repair of the immune system has to date been considered the least important aspect of treatment and control of these infections. There is developing evidence that support of the immune system is possible in these patients. Therefore, the effect of DMG on the immune system may be of benefit in immunosuppressive disorders."

Quercetin

Quercetin is a bioflavonoid found in onions, broccoli, and squash that is a potent anticancer nutrient and membrane stabilizer. Quercetin is a potent inhibitor of bowel cancer. It is also protective against heart disease.

TABLE 12.1
Protection against Cancer

Nutrient	Daily Amount
Beta-carotene	10,000–30,000 IU
Vitamin A*	5,000–25,000 IU
Vitamin E	100–400 IU
Vitamin C	1,500–12,000 mg
Selenium	100–200 mcg
Pycnogenol	50–150 mg
Glutathione	as per label
Cysteine	500–1500 mg
Fiber	see Chapter 14
EPA (fish oil)	as per label
GLA (evening primrose oil)	as per label
Calcium	500–750 mg
Vitamin D	100–400 IU
Vitamin B-complex	as per label
Dimethylglycine (DMG)	100–200 mg
Quercetin	100–300 mg

*If beta-carotene is taken, less vitamin A is required. The range therefore would be 5,000 to 15,000 IU.

Supplements

Those concerned about their risk of cancer may wish to consider supplementing their diet. Reasonable levels of supplements to consider are listed in Table 12.1.

There is no such thing as 100% protection or guarantee against cancer, but optimal nutrition will offer you greater protection against cancer than being suboptimally nourished.

13

Preventing Lung Cancer

This section is primarily for smokers, but nonsmokers breathing a great deal of secondhand smoke can also benefit from this section. Also, many people live in homes where the radon level is dangerously high and may cause lung cancer.

Each year the number of adult smokers declines. Everyone is aware of the health hazards linked to smoking. You've seen them hundreds of times, so there is no need to list them again. Yet you still smoke! And you will until you decide to stop. You can't be scared into quitting. You may even want to stop, but so far you haven't been able to stop. Maybe the next time you try, or soon after that, you will be successful. Or maybe you enjoy smoking so much that you wouldn't want to deprive yourself, no matter what the danger might be. The question is not whether you should or will stop smoking, but what you can do to protect yourself from adverse effects while you do smoke.

The good news is that you can reduce your risk of cancer and heart disease to levels lower than average. The "prudent" advice is that you give up smoking. That's good advice, but useless if you have decided to ignore it or find that you can't follow it at this time. The prudent advice is not the best advice anyway. The best advice is to give up smoking and protect yourself against cancer and heart disease with the "alternative" strategy. Unfortunately, too many people follow the prudent advice and are unaware of the new research that supports the alternative advice.

Figure 13.1 shows that smokers getting adequate vitamin A and/or its starting material, beta-carotene, have less lung cancer than nonsmokers consuming less vitamin A and/or beta-carotene. Figure 13.1 analyzes three variables: beta-carotene intake, number of years of smoking, and the incidence of cancer. The figure shows the three variables in three dimensions, which gives us a format of twelve smaller squares forming a larger square. At two corners of the larger square are the two expected extremes: (a) The greatest cancer incidence is among those persons consuming the least amount of beta-carotene and smoking the longest; and (b) the lowest cancer incidence—actually zero—is among those eating the most beta-carotene and not smoking.[1]

However, many people were surprised by the data shown

Figure 13.1

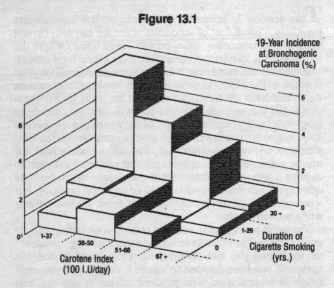

From Dietary Vitamin A and Risk of Cancer in the Western Electric study, Shekelle, Richard B, et al., The Lancet 1185-9 (Nos. 28, 1981).

by the remaining two corners of the larger square. Those nonsmokers eating little beta-carotene had a slightly higher incidence of cancer than those who had been smoking for more than thirty years but were getting adequate beta-carotene. That's correct—beta-carotene is a better protector against cancer than not smoking!

In the group of thirty-year smokers, the cancer incidence decreases with increasing beta-carotene in the diet from a 6.5% cancer rate for the lowest level (100–3,700 IU of beta-carotene) to a 4.5% cancer rate for 3,800–5,000 IU (the conservative "official" recommended dietary allowance is 5,000 IU total beta-carotene and vitamin A, but the RDA doesn't consider cancer protection), to a 3.0% cancer rate for the 5,100–6,600 IU group, to 0.8% for those eating more than 6,700 IU of beta-carotene daily.

Among those smoking from one to twenty-nine years, the cancer incidence falls with increasing beta-carotene consumption, but the difference is not as great because fewer years have passed to allow the cancer to form. The cancer incidence is 2.5% for the lowest beta-carotene level, 2.4% for the 3,800–5,000 IU group, and about 0.4% for the two highest beta-carotene groups.

Among the nonsmokers, the cancer incidence is 0.9% for the lowest beta-carotene group, 2.4% for the group getting just less than the RDA, about one percent for those getting just more than the RDA, and absolutely zero percent for those getting the most beta-carotene.

Some of the increase found in the nonsmoking group may be accounted for by two factors: Some nonsmokers breathe more secondhand smoke from their family members and co-workers than other nonsmokers, and some nonsmokers may be considerably older than most of those in the group smoking only one to twenty-nine years.

Note that at all levels of beta-carotene intake, the cancer rate was lower in the nonsmoking group than in the corresponding thirty-year-plus smoking group. The surprise is in the comparison of smokers eating lots of beta-carotene to nonsmokers eating little beta-carotene, as explained above.

Merely by optimizing your dietary intake of vitamin A and beta-carotene you can lower your risk of cancer. But there is more that you can do, because other nutrients are also protective.

Figure 13.1 is not a hypothetical illustration. It represents data from a nineteen-year study of 1,954 men. However, that is not our only hard evidence. Dr. Regina Ziegler of the National Cancer Institute studied over 1,000 people and found that these nutrients measurably counteracted the effects of exposure to cancer-causing agents like tobacco (ACS meeting, Daytona, April, 1984).

Other epidemiological studies support these findings. Earlier in 1980 Dr. N. Wald's group published an epidemiological study that attracted the interest of Dr. Shekelle's group.[2] Two other studies also showed that low levels of vitamin A in the blood were associated with high incidence of lung cancer.[3,4]

This is not really surprising. Researchers first noticed in 1925 that there was a relationship between a deficiency in vitamin A and cancer. Several experiments from the 1930s through the 1950s confirmed this relationship. Since then we have learned that cancer-causing chemicals can react strongly with DNA in vitamin A–deficient cells, that cancers are hard to transplant into animals adequately nourished with vitamin A, and that vitamin A is therapeutic in dealing with precancerous cells.

Vitamin A deficiency prevents a mucous coating from forming on the trachea, lungs, rectum, digestive system, and the inside of the skin. The vitamin A deficiency isn't the cause of cancer, but it makes these areas less resistant to cancer.

In one of Dr. Umberto Saffioti's experiments when he was at the Chicago Medical School (he later joined the National Cancer Institute), 113 hamsters were dosed with the cancer-causing chemical in cigarette smoke, benzopyrene. In the 53 control animals not given *extra* vitamin A protection, 16 developed lung cancer. However, in the 60 vitamin A–treated animals, only one developed cancer.

Dr. E. Bjelke of the Cancer Registry of Norway found that 74% of men with lung cancer were in the lowest third of the population ranked by vitamin A intake. He also found that vitamin-deficient city dwellers have three times the lung cancer rate of better-nourished city dwellers.

These studies agree well with the beta-carotene studies illustrated in Figure 13.1. Beta-carotene is converted to vitamin A in the body, but it has its own protective action as well.

Never will the alternative strategy alone give you better health than combining nonsmoking with the alternative strategy, but it can be better than just nonsmoking alone.

The preachers of good health—those holier than thou—insist that you quit smoking, or you can just go to hell. Well, you may just get the last laugh, if you protect yourself as much as possible now, and live to a distant day when you may or may not decide to join the "prudent" group—if they are still around.

Radon in the Home Causes Lung Cancer

Radon is believed to be the third or fourth leading cause of lung cancer. Figures in the December 1988 issue of the *New England Journal of Medicine* estimate that smoking causes 130,200 deaths from lung cancer each year, secondhand smoke is responsible for between 2,500 and 8,400 lung cancer deaths each year, about 5,000 lung cancer deaths may be caused by asbestos, and up to 4,700 lung cancer deaths are due to radon. The Environmental Protection Agency estimates between 5,000 and 20,000 lung cancer deaths each year are due to radon. A 1988 National Academy of Sciences study estimates that radon causes 13,000 lung cancer deaths yearly. It is hoped that both the EPA and NAS estimates are high.

Radon is a radioactive gas that accumulates in homes from certain soils. Radon's radioactivity initiates free radicals that cause cancer. Radon is a neutral gas in terms of chemical reactivity, but it is highly radioactive. It arises from the radioactive decay of uranium. Traces of uranium are found in gravel and in many rocks throughout the nation.

Of course, in the Southwest, where there are large concentrations of uranium, the radon problem is a major concern. However, even in the East, rock formations of granite, shale, and phosphates have enough uranium to produce significant amounts of radon. Since radon is a gas, it seeps up through cracks in the bedrock and soil and can be trapped within a tightly sealed home. When the concentration in the air builds to a certain level, the risk of lung cancer increases. Just what that "critical level" is remains to be established at this writing. The EPA and the various states are debating the issue, and the evidence is scanty at best.

However, the fact that radon causes lung cancer in humans is well established. The fact that miners have a high incidence of lung disease has been known since 1556. (That's not a typo—1556.) The disease was recognized as lung cancer as early as 1879. At the turn of the century it was killing about one half of U.S. mine workers. It wasn't until the 1950s and 1960s that epidemiological studies confirmed that radon was the culprit.

Radon gets its name from radium. Uranium-238 slowly decays radioactively to produce radium-226 and other by-products, with the radium radioactively decaying to produce radon-222 and other by-products. The radon releases alpha-radiation but lasts only a relatively short time (half-life of radon-222 is 3.8 days). The problem is the decay products of radon. The decay products are called radon progeny. The radon progeny are solids and tend to lodge in the lungs. Some of the radon progeny have very long radioactive lifetimes.

The antioxidant nutrients offer protection against the free radicals produced in the lungs by radon progeny. However, it is still prudent to have your home and workplace tested to determine their radon levels. The EPA estimates that nearly 20,000,000 homes are poisoned with radon, but the exact number will depend on the level that is finally agreed upon as being critical. Test kits are widely available, but check with your local or state health office for recommendations.

Lung Protection

A combination of antioxidant nutrients is necessary to protect the lungs against cancer. It makes no difference if the causative agent is smoke or radon. Let's review the main antioxidant nutrients as they pertain to lung cancer.

Vitamin A and Beta-carotene

As discussed earlier, vitamin A protects the lungs in several ways. If a person is deficient in vitamin A, changes can occur in the lung tissues that encourage cancer formation—even without an overwhelming exposure to cigarette smoke or radon. Vitamin A–deficient cells in the lungs can be easily mutated by chemicals normally present in the air.

Vitamin A also is an antioxidant, which means that vitamin A sacrifices itself by reacting with pollutants in such a way as to protect the cells from the pollutants.

Vitamin A may also help "direct" cell growth. Immature cells can become one of several types of mature cells. Vitamin A may help determine if an immature cell growing in a bronchial tube becomes either a mucous cell or a cilia cell. Vitamin A may also help keep a damaged cell from growing abnormally.

Beta-carotene is converted in the body to vitamin A; thus, beta-carotene does all the good things that vitamin A does, plus it does what only beta-carotene can do. The unique property of beta-carotene is that it can destroy a particularly harmful form of oxygen called "singlet oxygen." Singlet oxygen is often found in polluted air and cigarette smoke.

As the body uses up its supply of vitamin A more beta-carotene is converted into vitamin A. However, too much oxidizing air pollution or cigarette smoke can destroy vitamin A so rapidly that little protection is given to the lung cells no matter how much vitamin A or beta-carotene is in the diet. This is because the vitamin A is stored in the liver and must be transported to the lungs in a special protein called retinol-binding protein.

This is where other antioxidants such as vitamin E and selenium become important. The other antioxidants also sacrifice themselves to the pollutants, and, as a bonus, they protect molecules of vitamin A so that they can reach the lung cells. The other antioxidants are not limited by the retinol-binding protein transport system. Therefore, a combination of antioxidant nutrients is synergistic in protecting the lungs.

There are multiple pathways in which the chemicals that cause cancer can do their damage. However, all of the pathways can be blocked by the antioxidant nutrients vitamins A, C, and E, plus the trace mineral selenium. These nutrients protect the cell from penetration by the cancer-causing chemicals; they prevent the chemicals from reacting with the cell and DNA (the "life" compound that reproduces body components); and they stimulate your natural immunity to cancer. Even if a cancer develops in the body, it can be destroyed by your immune system—if your immune system is not impaired by suboptimal nutrition.

Vitamin C

Vitamin C is more than an antioxidant. It also prevents nitrates in the stomach from being converted into cancer-causing nitrosamines. Of importance to smokers is that vitamin C can prevent damaging reactions with acetaldehyde and other chemicals in smoke or produced by smoke.[5] Vitamin C is known to protect against more than fifty pollutants. Unfortunately, smoking lowers the amount of vitamin C in the blood. Smokers must consume more vitamin C than nonsmokers to have the same amount in their blood.

Vitamin C also stimulates the immune system. Specifically, vitamin C stimulates the production of lymphocytes and interferon.[6] Epidemiological studies by Dr. Bjelke and others show that cancer is high when vitamin C is low and vice versa.

Further details are found in "Cancer and Vitamin C" by Drs. Ewan Cameron and Linus Pauling. (Norton & Co., NY 1979)

Vitamin E

Low levels of vitamin E are also associated with increased risk of lung cancer.[7,8]

At a 1989 conference on vitamin E conducted by the New

York Academy of Sciences, Dr. Garry Duthe of Rowett Research Institute in Aberdeen, Scotland confirmed that vitamin E prevented the buildup of free radicals in smokers. He and his colleagues compared the red blood cells of twenty male smokers with those of twenty male nonsmokers. Then they gave half of each group 1,000 IU daily for two weeks. The others took placebos. They found that the red blood cells of the smokers receiving the placebo were three times more susceptible to free radical damage. *But the red blood cells of the smokers who were given vitamin E were as resistant to free-radical damage as were those of nonsmokers.*

Selenium was shown to be safe and protective against lung cancer at 300 micrograms daily in a Chinese study.[9] A Finnish study confirmed that there is an inverse relationship between the amount of selenium in the blood and the risk of cancer.[10]

Folic Acid

Dr. Douglas Heimburger and colleagues at the University of Alabama Medical Center found that folic acid helps prevent lung injury from smoking. They studied seventy-three male heavy smokers and found that fourteen of thirty-six volunteers given folic acid and vitamin B-12 supplements had reduced lung injury after four months. In the placebo control group, six of thirty-seven spontaneously improved.[11]

Other Dietary Factors

There is even an additional system in which the diet can protect against cancer. (By the way, if you are unconvinced that diet is related to cancer, just study the change in cancer incidence that occurs when a group of people changes its dietary habits—such as Japanese and Africans adopting Western diets.) Certain nutrients can bind to chemicals that cause cancer or convert them to harmless compounds.

One example involves benzo(a)pyrene, (BP), the chemical in cigarette smoke that causes cancer. Well, actually, BP is not the chemical that does the harm. It is the chemical that gets into the body via smoke but then is converted by enzymes called aryl hydrocarbon hydroxylases into a more potent chemical that is the epoxide of BP. The chemistry is not important to understand, but it may help you understand why not everyone who inhales BP gets cancer.

Some people have more of the enzymes that convert BP into the cancer-causing epoxide than other people. Thus they make larger amounts of the epoxide in their bodies in a shorter time, thus producing a greater concentration of the BP epoxide.

On the other hand, BP and its epoxide can be bound by the nutrient glutathione and thus rendered harmless. A diet rich in glutathione is protective against cancer. It is also interesting to note that one study has been published in *Science* (May, 1981) showing that glutathione supplements cured liver cancer in laboratory animals.

The amino acid cysteine detoxifies compounds produced in the body by the act of smoking. These compounds are called aldehydes, and they cause injury to body cells. Aldehydes are believed to cross-link healthy cells together in such a way as to impair their function. Although aldehydes may not be a direct cause of lung cancer, they do damage that impairs the body's defenses and prematurely ages the skin. The nutrient cysteine (L-cysteine) should be in your defense arsenal.

Supplements

Those concerned about their risk of lung cancer may wish to consider supplementing their diet. Reasonable levels of supplements to consider are listed in Table 13.1. The "prudent" advice, of course, is not to expose the body tissues to cigarette smoke and radon in the first place. This time the "alternative" approach would come out second best if it were not for the fact that most people are not living under ideal conditions. They are exposed to other pollutants that can cause

TABLE 13.1
Protection against Lung Cancer

Nutrient	Amount
Beta-carotene	10,000–30,000 IU
Vitamin A*	5,000–25,000 IU
Vitamin E	100–400 IU
Vitamin C	1,500–12,000 mg
Selenium	100–200 mcg
Glutathione	as per label
Cysteine	500–1500 mg
Folic Acid	400–800 mcg
Vitamin B-12	50–100 mcg

*If beta-carotene is taken, less vitamin A is required. The range therefore would be 5,000 to 15,000 IU.

lung cancer, and they are not optimally nourished. As the evidence shows, a well-nourished smoker is at less risk than those that are poorly nourished living in our contaminated environment.

14

Preventing Colon Cancer

Colon cancer is the nation's second most common cancer, striking about 150,000 persons each year and killing 60,000. High-fat, low-fiber diets are thought of as risk factors in heart disease, but more important, they are definite risk factors in colon (bowel) cancer. Dr. Bruce Trock reviewed thirty-seven studies and concluded that eating more vegetables, fruits, and grains would lower a person's risk of colon cancer by 40%. The thirty-seven studies he reviewed involved more than 10,000 people in fifteen countries. [*J. Nat. Cancer Inst.*, 1990] Protection against heart disease is relatively simple, but extra measures must be taken to protect against bowel cancer.

Typical American diets are high in fat, low in fiber, and low in nutrition. Yet that is what most Americans choose to eat. Nutrition and health are secondary to "good eating," which to most is the good taste of traditional meals. Vegetarians have little risk of colon cancer, while those eating red meat daily have 2.5 times the risk of colon cancer as vegetarians. Of course, the "prudent" people heed the warnings and switch to low-fat, high-fiber meals. It seems that the vast majority, however, would rather be dead than to eat all that tasteless rabbit food and grains.

Many of the brave who are willing to try a low-fat, high-fiber diet soon abandon it for one reason or another. If you are one of the lucky ones who enjoy a low-fat, high-fiber diet, congratulations; skip on to another chapter that interests you. However, if you are one of the great majority, read on to learn how you can protect yourself against the cancer-promoting action of excess fat and low fiber.

The antioxidant nutrients discussed in the preceding chapter are protective against excess fats, but an extra step is required to reduce the risk induced by a lack of fiber. The good news is that you can protect yourself without changing your diet, but the bad news is that it is not quite as simple as taking a pill. Let's see what's involved.

Colon Cancer

Cancer of the colon (large intestine or bowel) appears to be caused by two primary mechanisms. The first is the ingestion of certain chemicals that will directly cause bowel cancer. Although this is produced at will in laboratory animals, it is hardly ever the case with people, because such chemicals are rarely ingested in sufficient quantities over a sufficient period of time except in industrial situations.

The normal mechanism in human bowel cancer seems to be the increased absorption of chemicals through the walls of the bowel. The increased absorption of harmful chemicals is caused by prolonged exposure to these chemicals due to their remaining in the bowel abnormally long. The abnormal length of stay in the bowel is a result of a lack of fiber, which serves the purpose of stimulating the bowel muscles to push things along.

The chemicals involved can be normal carcinogens that may be consumed in the diet, but most often they are the breakdown products of bile and fats. Normally, when a high-fiber diet is consumed, the bile and fats are pushed through the system before they putrefy or degrade.

A high-fiber diet normally produces a transit time through the body of one or two days. The food consumed by Africans eating their normal tribal diets travels from the mouth through the body in one day. In contrast, the food consumed by the average Westerner requires at least three days for the same trip. Indeed, many low-fiber diets require up to two weeks to be eliminated.

Even if an individual on such a low-fiber diet maintains bowel regularity, the fecal matter containing bile and leftover digestion products remains in the bowel to putrefy or turn rancid, and these harmful chemicals are in contact with the bowel membranes for days.

New Discovery

Scientists have recently discovered that when the bacteria normally present in the bowel die they decompose, yielding the very powerful cancer-causing substance fecapentaene (a shortened version of its longer chemical name).[1] The more fiber in the diet, the healthier the bacteria and the less fecapentaene. In addition, the two main components of bile are the bile acids, cholic acid and deoxycholic acid. If bile is allowed to slosh around in the bowel for a while, bacteria will convert the cholic acid into the proven cancer-causer apcholic acid, and the deoxycholic acid will be converted into one of the most dangerous cancer-producers known, 3-MCA (3-methyl-cholanthrene).

Also, bacteria can change relatively harmless chemicals and drugs into potent carcinogens. Another point of interest is that people eating a high-fiber diet have mostly "good" bacteria, lactobacillus and streptococcus, while those eating low-fiber diets harbor mostly "bad" bacteria, bifidobacteria and bacteroides. The "good" bacteria do not degrade bile, fats, and other chemicals into compounds that cause cancer, whereas the "bad" bacteria do.

Scientists noted that the Finns, who eat a Western diet abundant in beef, fat, and protein and low in fiber, have a relatively low incidence of colon cancer. They also eat a relatively large amount of yogurt and have been shown to harbor large numbers of lactobacilli in their intestines.[2]

Clinical studies have shown that when large amounts of *L. acidophilus* are taken orally, the enzymes that degrade intestinal matter into cancer-causing substances are greatly diminished. In studies where laboratory animals were given chemicals known to cause colon cancer, those animals also fed large amounts of *L. acidophilus* had relatively little colon cancer.

Those who eat low-fiber diets tend to have bacteria that produce cancer-causing chemicals and also have a slow transit time that keeps these chemicals in contact with their bowels for long periods. But it doesn't have to be that way! High-fat diets compound the problem by supplying excess fats that escape digestion and absorption and find their way into the colon, where they are oxidized and produce the harmful free radicals discussed in previous chapters.

However, low-fiber, high-fat diets are a problem in regard to bowel cancer only when the transit time through the bowel is slow. The question then becomes, "How does one know what his or her transit time is?"

Measuring Your Transit Time

Your first concern, then, is to determine if you have a slow transit time that puts you at excessive risk. You can easily measure your transit time by using a stool marker such as charcoal tablets. The charcoal will pass through your body in the same time that your food residues will pass through. After taking four to six charcoal tablets, observe your feces until you note the appearance of the charcoal.

If your transit time exceeds two days, then you should be concerned about protecting yourself from the risk of bowel cancer. If your transit time is more than four days, you should be aggressive in taking the protective steps.

Protection

The problems due to fats reaching the colon can be controlled with antioxidant nutrients that protect the fats from oxidation and destroy free radicals that might be produced. The longer the fats remain in the bowel, the more they need the protection of the antioxidant nutrients.

The high-fiber diet of Africans contains about 25 grams of fiber daily. The average Western diet contains about 8 grams. The difference is only an average of 17 grams, or about three quarters of an ounce.[3] American vegetarians apparently get adequate fiber.

A one-ounce cup of all-bran cereal will give you about 9 grams of fiber; one third cup of baked beans will provide about 7 grams; one third cup of spinach will contain about 4 grams; a medium apple about three-and-a-half grams; and a slice of whole wheat bread contains about 2 grams of fiber.

Rather than adding a specified amount of fiber to your diet, you should consider adding fiber until your transit time becomes less than two days, or until your stools float. You should also be sure to drink adequate fluids to swell up the undigested fiber in your bowel to produce the desired soft-but-firm bulk. Additionally, you should be sure you are getting adequate mineral intakes, because extra fiber may carry out some minerals bound to the fiber.

There are two main physical categories of fiber—soluble and insoluble—and five chemical classes of fibers—cellulose, hemicelluloses, gums, pectin, and lignin—and you should have ample amounts of each in your diet.

Soluble fibers can help lower high blood cholesterol levels, and insoluble fibers can decrease transit time.

Celluloses increase bulk, soften stools, relieve constipation, counteract bowel carcinogens, modulate blood sugar levels, and help control appetite. Celluloses have no known effect on blood cholesterol levels. Excellent sources are fruits, vegetables, bran, seeds, nuts, and beans.

Hemicelluloses increase bulk, relieve constipation, counteract bowel carcinogens, and help control appetite. Their effects are very similar to cellulose, and they are found in the same foods.

Gums lower blood cholesterol and modulate blood sugar levels. Good food sources of gums are oats, barley, and dried beans. Pectins lower blood cholesterol, counter bowel bile acids, and offer some protection against bowel cancer and gallstones. Gums and pectins are water-soluble and thus do not hold water. Therefore they have no effect on stool bulk and constipation. Good food sources for pectins are carrots, apples, prunes, citrus fruits, and, contrary to popular opinion, bran.

Lignins increase removal of cholesterol and bile acids from the bowel, thereby protecting against bowel cancer and gallstones. Good sources are prunes, cereals, bran, fruits, and vegetables.

Whole grains, vegetables, and fruits are excellent fiber sources. Bran and vegetable fiber supplements are available that can be added to your favorite foods, mixed with juices, or chewed as tablets.

Table 14.1 is a guide to which foods have which types of fiber.

TABLE 14.1
Fibers and Their Effects

Good Cancer Protection (Insoluble Fiber)	(Both)	Good Heart Protection (Soluble Fiber)
Wheat bran	Kidney beans	Apples
Wheat products	Navy beans	Bananas
Brown rice	Green beans	Citrus fruits
Cooked lentils	Green peas	Carrots
	Pinto beans	Barley
		Oats
		Rice bran

Acidophilus

You can encourage the "good" bacteria to persist in your bowel over the "bad" bacteria by taking *Lactobacillus acidophilus* supplements, drinking acidophilus milk, or eating yogurt (L. bulgarius).

Calcium

Drs. Cedrick Garland and Frank Garland of the University of California at San Diego became intrigued with the geographic pattern of bowel cancer incidence. They noted that there was much less bowel cancer in the southern "sunshine" states. Their studies led them to conclude that the extra vitamin D produced in the skin of those receiving greater sun exposure in the southern states aided calcium absorption. Further studies of calcium intake and bowel cancer supported the theory that calcium helps protect against bowel cancer.[4]

As a follow-up of the epidemiological findings, Drs. Martin Lipkin and Harold Newmark of the Sloan-Kettering Cancer Center studied the effect of 1,250 milligrams of calcium per day on persons in families that have a history of bowel cancer. They found that after three months these persons at high risk for bowel cancer had a normalization of rate of intestinal cell division.[5,6]

Selenium

Dr. Clark Griffin of the M. D. Anderson Hospital and Tumor Institute in Houston showed that selenium was protective against bowel cancer in laboratory animals given three different chemicals that cause bowel cancer. Dr. Charles Shaw, a member of the M. D. Anderson group, showed that selenium alone reduced bowel cancer from 87% to 40% in his laboratory animal studies.

Vitamin C

In a study of fifty-eight patients with a high risk of developing bowel cancer due to a family history (familial adenomatous polyposis), four grams of vitamin C plus 400 IU of vitamin E daily, along with a high-fiber diet, produced a greater decline in polyps than a high-fiber diet without the added vitamins.[7]

Quercetin

Quercetin is a bioflavonoid found in onions, broccoli, and squash that is a potent anticancer nutrient and membrane stabilizer. Quercetin is especially protective against bowel cancer.

Supplements

Consult Table 14.2 for diet supplements to help normalize your transit time and to reduce undesirable degradation. Don't forget that you can combine the "prudent" and "alternative" strategies for even better health. Try adding more vegetables and fruits to your present diet. You could see more benefits, such as weight normalization and better digestion.

TABLE 14.2
Protection against Colon Cancer

Nutrient	Daily Amount
Bran or other fiber supplement	10 grams
Acidophilus *(Lactobacillus acidophilus)*	1 capsule
Vitamin E	100–400 IU
Vitamin C	1,250–12,000 mg
Vitamin A or beta-carotene	10,000–20,000 IU
Calcium	750–1,000 mg
Zinc	15–25 mg
Quercetin	250–750 mg

15

Preventing Breast and Cervical Cancers

———————■———————

The number and rate of breast cancer deaths are increasing. Breast cancer is the second leading cause of female cancer deaths. It killed 40,354 women in the U.S. in 1986. The annual death rate for 1986 was 32.8 per 100,000 women, which was up five percent from 1979. Breast cancer is striking 115,000 American women each year, a rate that will affect one in every twelve women.

Yet the evidence indicates that breast cancer can be reduced more dramatically than any other cancer, thanks to antioxidants. This promising and strong evidence may be the reason there are so many studies on the subject.

Selenium

An early clue came from a study by Drs. Raymond Shamberger and Douglas Frost of the level of selenium in crops and the rate of breast cancer in various areas. Below a certain level of selenium, the incidence of breast cancer dramatically increases above the average rate, and this increase is inversely proportional to selenium level. When selenium exceeds this level, the breast cancer rate is 20% below average.

Additional studies confirmed that breast cancer rate was also *inversely* proportional to blood selenium levels.[1]

In 1976 Dr. Christine Wilson, a nutritionist at the University of California at San Francisco, reported her study showing that high-selenium diets protected against breast cancer. After comparing the nutrient content of an average non-Western diet supplying 2,500 calories to that of a typical American diet providing the same number of calories, Dr. Wilson determined that the Western diets contained about a fourth of the selenium of the Asian diets. Also significant was the presence of more "easily oxidizable" polyunsaturated fat (7.5 to 8.7 grams a day) than in the Western diets (10 to 30 grams).

The combination of high selenium and low polyunsaturated fats may be protecting Asian women against breast cancer.[2]

A dramatic laboratory-animal study supports this hypothesis. The incidence of spontaneous breast cancer in susceptible female mice was reduced from 82% to 10% merely by adding selenium to their diet. The study was conducted by Dr. Gerhard Schrauzer of the University of California at San Diego in 1974.[3]

Besides the eightfold reduction in cancer incidence, there were other important benefits achieved. In the 10% that did develop cancer, the tumors did not appear until 50% later than among the control animals, and the tumors were "less malignant."

Dr. Schrauzer believes that if a breast cancer patient has especially low selenium blood levels, her tendency to develop metastases is increased, her possibility for survival is diminished, and her outlook in general is poorer than if she has a normal blood selenium level.

On several occasions Dr. Schrauzer has told me that he firmly believes that the key to cancer prevention lies in assuring the adequate intake of selenium, as well as other essential trace elements.

Dr. Schrauzer claims, "If every woman in America started taking selenium supplements or had a high-selenium diet, then within a few years the breast cancer rate in this country would drastically decline."

Epidemiological studies of twenty-seven countries comparing their selenium intake and breast cancer rate also indicate that selenium is protective. Figures 15.1 and 15.2 show these relationships.

Vitamin E

Dr. N. J. Wald of the Medical College of St. Bartholomew's Hospital in London published a report showing that *women in the lowest fifth of blood vitamin E levels had five times the breast cancer rate of women in the highest fifth.*[4]

Vitamin A

Dr. Gregory Hislop and his colleagues at the Cancer Control Agency of British Columbia studied 450 breast cancer patients and concluded, "Vitamin A supplements and frequent consumption of green vegetables—often rich in beta-carotene and other carotenoids—appear to protect women against the more proliferate breast disease, apparently lowering a woman's breast cancer risk by more than half."[5] Even heavy consumption of fat did not appear to influence the development of this abnormality, though it did increase the risk of developing severe atypias. (Fat will be discussed later.) Dr. Hislop concluded, "Vitamin A may play a role in the earlier stages of [precancerous] disease, and dietary fat later on."

B Complex

The degree to and rate at which the female sex hormone estrogen is converted into estradiol is thought by some researchers to be linked to breast cancer. The number of receptors for these compounds in breast tissue may also be involved. Adequate nourishment with several members of the

Figure 15.1

Zero cancer extrapolations

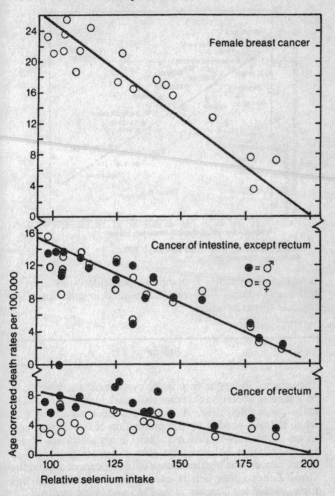

Source: Schrauzer, White, and Schneider, 1977. *Bioinorganic Chem.* 7:37.

Figure 15.2

Relationship of selenium intake and breast cancer mortalities

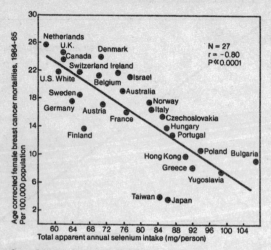

Source: Schrauzer, G., White, D. and Schneider, C. 1977.
Bioinorganic Chemistry, vol. 7, p. 36.

family of the vitamin B complex—particularly choline, inositol and vitamin B-6—and the mineral magnesium helps
regulate this conversion.

Iodine

The mineral iodine helps prevent cystic mastitis, which can
be a painful condition that can also mask lumps and prevent
early cancer detection. A theory has been advanced that
when iodine—needed for the production of the thyroid hormone thyroxine—is deficient there is an alteration of estrogen-estradiol balance, and thus a greater incidence of
breast cancer. The high incidence of breast cancer around the
Great Lakes goiter belt is cited. For a discussion of this
topic, please see Chapter 24 on PMS and cystic mastitis.

Diet

Fat and total calories have also been linked to breast cancer in some studies but not confirmed in others. In postmenopausal women dietary fat can influence the production of estrogen and the estrogen-estradiol balance. In premenopausal women the normal production of estrogen is not affected as much by dietary fat. Dr. Ross Prentice of the Fred Hutchinson Cancer Research Center in Seattle found that low-fat diets reduced the blood levels of estradiol.[6]

As Dr. Wilson pointed out earlier in this chapter, dietary fat and body fat can become sources of free radicals that can cause cancer. Cutting back on fat and total calories may help reduce the amount of free radicals, but antioxidant nutrients are still required to protect whatever fats do exist in the body.

Several studies have confirmed that women who drink alcohol are at increased risk of breast cancer. The increase in risk is proportional to the amount of alcohol consumed.

"The Pill" and Estrogen Replacement

As I said in *Supernutrition*, the long-term use of some birth-control pills is still linked to increased risk of breast cancer in younger women. The number of women affected may not be extremely large because breast cancer is fairly uncommon in younger women. The British study led by Dr. Julian Peto of the Institute of Cancer Research in London was published in May, 1989 in *Lancet*.[7]

Dr. Peto and his colleagues found a 70% increase in breast cancer risk among women under age thirty-six who took the pill for at least eight years. They found a 40% increase among those women who took the pill for four to eight years.

Newer birth control pills that are lower in dosage may not produce this effect. The pill also reduced the risk for ovarian and uterine cancer.

A Swedish study casts some doubt on the safety of replacement hormone therapy for postmenopausal women. Although only two of thirty studies show a link between estrogen replacement therapy and breast cancer, it is a matter of concern. The Swedish study is discussed in Chapter 9 on menopause.

Preventing Cervical Cancer

A deficiency of the nutrient folic acid (also called folacin) causes cell changes that lead to cervical cancer. Folic acid deficiency causes abnormal cells to form in the cervix. These cells can be detected by a Pap smear. These abnormal cells are considered premalignant, but fortunately, they can be restored to normality by correcting the folic acid deficiency.

Also, the use of some birth-control pills can cause the abnormal cells to form even when adequate folic acid is eaten in the diet. In this case, taking extra folic acid supplements will usually restore the cells to normal.[8–11]

A deficiency of vitamin A or beta-carotene increases the incidence of cervical cancer. As discussed in Chapter 13 on lung cancer, vitamin A is critical in producing normal mucous membrane cells. Vitamin A helps epithelial cells mature and differentiate.

Whatever causes cervical cells to change can be stopped by vitamin A. Some researchers are investigating the possibility that a virus called human papilloma virus (HPV) causes changes in cervical cells that can lead to cancer. Vitamin A and beta-carotene can stop the growth of cells infected with HPV, according to Dr. Kim Creek of the University of South Carolina.

Australian researchers compared the blood levels of vitamin A and beta-carotene and the diets of 117 cervical cancer patients with those of 196 matched controls. They found no relationship with vitamin A and cervical cancer risk, but a strong correlation with low beta-carotene levels and cervical cancer risk.[10,11] Women in the highest quarter of beta-carotene intake had only one fifth the incidence of cervical cancer of those in the lowest quarter.

They also found a relationship between low vitamin C intake and cervical cancer incidence. Women in the highest quarter of vitamin C intake had only 60% of the cervical cancer incidence of those in the lowest quarter.

A confirming study was reported by a University of Utah group. Dr. M. Slattery and colleagues found protective effects for vitamins A, C, and E and beta-carotene.[12]

Similar findings were reported by an Italian research team. They compared the diets of 392 women with cervical cancer to the diets of 392 matched controls. They found that women consuming less than 5,000 IU daily of vitamin A and/or beta-carotene had three times the incidence of cervical cancer of those consuming more. Those women who averaged less than 3,000 IU daily had five times the incidence of cervical cancer.[13]

Supplements

Consult Table 15.1 for a list of supplements that women should especially consider.

TABLE 15.1
Protection against Breast and Cervical Cancers

Nutrient	Daily Amount
Selenium	200 mcg
Kelp (iodine)	one tablet daily
Magnesium	250–500 mg
Vitamin A	5,000–10,000 IU
Beta-carotene	5,000–15,000 IU
Vitamin C	1,250–11,000 mg
Vitamin E	400–600 IU
B-complex	one capsule daily
Folic acid	800 mcg
Evening primrose oil (GLA)	one capsule daily

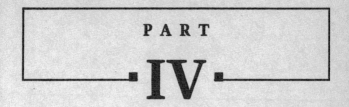

PART

· IV ·

Supernutrition Against Heart Disease

16

Heart Disease Causes

———————— ■ ————————

Believe it or not, there is still a raging debate as to whether or not dietary cholesterol is a cause of high blood cholesterol resulting in heart disease. Let's not put all of our eggs in one basket. You can choose your side, or you can follow the best advice of both sides. I will present both sides, and you can do as you please.

As I discussed extensively in *Supernutrition*, I don't believe that the dietary-cholesterol proponents have scientifically proven their case, but that doesn't mean that it isn't so. Nature follows Nature's laws—not how well we design our experiments to learn Nature's laws. This chapter will discuss heart disease background and various theories of heart disease. The next chapter will show you how to lower your cholesterol by thirty points in thirty days, if you are concerned about cholesterol. The following chapter will show you how to prevent heart attacks regardless of your cholesterol level and the condition of your arteries.

Common advice is to stop smoking, exercise, and eat a low-fat, low-cholesterol, high-fiber diet. Sounds so simple, doesn't it? However, many people have chosen not to—or just plain can't—take these "prudent" steps! It would seem that if the prevailing advice happens to be correct, then these people have a higher risk of developing heart disease than they could have. But there is more than one route to achieving the goal of a healthy heart!

The dietary component of heart disease is not so much what you eat as it is what you don't eat. The vitamins and minerals that are missing from most diets are more important than the excess fats and cholesterol.

If the favorite techniques of conventional health professionals are not to your liking or are incompatible with your life-style, perhaps the "alternative" techniques may appeal to you. If you can't give up your favorite foods and cigarettes and are bored by jogging, maybe your style is to leisurely add a healthy food supplement or two to your meals. These lesser-known nutrients may be much more critical to heart health than the widely publicized and commercially touted nutritional approaches or exercise alone.

Most health professionals seem to believe that the only nutritional factors are the widely publicized ones, and that they are the only factors involved in heart disease other than activity, age, and heredity. Thus, most health advisors become upset at any approach that doesn't insist on low-fat, low-cholesterol, high-fiber meals plus exercise and abstinence from smoking.

Someday you may change to their "prudent" life-style. But why should you be thrown to the dogs just because you haven't fallen in step? Especially since there is another solution and even a happy medium. Don't you deserve some help now—before it's too late? With your improved health you may even become additionally motivated to make life-style changes later.

Of course, there is still the lingering question of whether marching to their drum is the best course of action for you. One man's meat is another man's poison. Dr. Roger Williams proved long ago that we are all somewhat biochemically unique.

Now for the great masses, there are few problems in following the "prudent" advice. That is, provided that it is not carried to extreme and that the adherents are well nourished. However, there may be danger for the trendy if they feel that their low-fat, low-cholesterol diets and exercise will fully protect them from heart disease. Even ardent supporters of these prudent practices will tell you that high cholesterol levels in the blood and a sedentary life-style will explain only half of the heart disease.

It may be that prudent measures are moderate factors for nearly all people, or major factors for a minor fraction of the population. If so, which subgroup of the population is affected by the prudent measures? And which by the "alternative" measures? Are more people affected by the direct control of the alternative measures? How many persons do you know that violate all of the prudent measures, yet are healthier and outlive nearly everyone else? Did these persons inherit strong genes, or have they been unknowingly following the alternative measures?

If eating rich, fatty foods, smoking, and lack of exercise were the only causes of heart disease, then prudent dieting, abstinence from smoking, and exercise would wipe heart disease off the map. Yet in those groups making the prudent changes, heart disease incidence hasn't been cut by anywhere near half. Now this is not to dismiss lightly cutting the heart disease rate in half. That's an admirable achievement.

But let's go after 100%—not 50%. Combining the prudent advice and the alternative advice may take us beyond the 50% reduction.

The point is that prudent measures do not produce 100% protection because they are not the primary factors, only indirect influences on body chemistry. You want to control body chemistry directly. A great deal of control can be achieved via the "alternative" measures, but greater control can be accomplished by combining both approaches.

We are not debating which approach works best for the majority or which approach works best for you as an individual. We are searching for the approach that you can live with and benefit from. It should be comforting to know that you have three choices: the "prudent" approach, the "alternative" approach, and the combination of both.

You should not feel that you are doomed just because of your life-style. You can add easy alternative health measures to your present life-style and outlive, outperform, and outenjoy many—if not most—of those who have made prudent changes.

Always keep in mind that you can do even better by taking both prudent and alternative measures. Maybe you can't make the prudent changes today, but you can reduce your risk now with the alternative measures, and since you will still be alive and well, you can then take the prudent steps whenever you wish.

The prime objective is to initiate the measures that are compatible with your life-style now!

Hardly a day goes by without the general public being informed of new studies that prove or cast doubt on the postulated link between diet and heart disease. However, the public—and many scientists as well—seems to hear only that information that reinforces what they already believe and that seems logical to them.

You can find any results you want in the literature to support any conclusion. Neither side seems to need more evidence. The views are mostly hardened. The majority of reports support one view, but science isn't decided by popular vote.

A wise medical pedagogue once stated, "I know that half of what I teach as fact will be proved false in ten years. The hard part is that I don't know which half." As Dr. Kenneth Brigham of Vanderbilt reminded us in the *New England Journal of Medicine*, "Both sides ought to know that telling the good guys from the bad guys is an exclusive function of history."

The scientific debate also interacts with commercialism. Cholesterolphobia is used to sell cereals over eggs, margarine over butter, soy over meat, and vegetable oil over lard.

Under what conditions are these influences beneficial to people, and under what conditions are they harmful? Proponents of the cholesterol theory believe that these are prudent steps even if dietary cholesterol and fats don't cause heart disease. They believe that there is enough evidence to make these prudent changes and that there is nothing to lose.

But are there dangers? Will all Americans be as healthy on such diets? Only if they also make sure that they get adequate vitamins and minerals. Is there a limit to any benefit in shifting from our recent meat-consumption pattern to more "moderate" meat consumption and then to more "stringent" diets? Will there be a decrease in assimilated micronutrients, and will that decrease produce more disease?

What would be the effect of cholesterol-lowering diets on persons already having optimal or low blood-cholesterol levels? Studies by Dr. Jay Kaplan of the Bowman Gray Medical School and Dr. Stephen Manuck of the University of Pittsburgh suggest that low-fat, low-cholesterol diets make monkeys more aggressive. They are 50% more likely to grab, bite, shove, and otherwise torment their neighbors. In clinical studies of those on low-fat, low-cholesterol diets or drugs that lower blood cholesterol levels there are more deaths due to violence and suicide.

Persons with gradually declining cholesterol levels are more likely to develop colon cancer. This has been shown *not* to be the result of the disease, but a possible factor in developing the disease. [*J. Amer. Med. Assoc.*, April 18, 1990)

What if the dietary cholesterol/fat approach to heart disease affects only a minor portion of the population, but the hoopla over this placates the population so much that interest and funds diminish and research is abandoned that might have found an approach that would prevent heart disease in the remainder of the population?

What if the multifactorial approach of reducing as many of the alleged "risk factors" as possible simultaneously is hindered, in that several of the changes are beneficial—e.g., reduced smoking, increased activity, reduced stress, optimized body weight—but the dietary changes are detrimental? Wouldn't this approach be helped by eliminating—rather than perpetuating—the harmful factor?

For all these reasons, it is imperative that we not depend on popular vote or intuition, but on hard science. Yet there are those who feel differently. They feel enough is known—let's save lives now. But what if their data don't reflect the real-world experience of healthy people?

Alternatives

Body chemistry is very complex and has several regulatory mechanisms to maintain chemical balance. The regulators adjust for changing conditions, including most dietary changes. In essence, if we eat balanced meals containing all of the food factors that we need in the appropriate amounts, then body chemistry is normal. However, if our diet gets out of balance, and we eat too much of some components and not enough of other components, body chemistry—and blood chemistry—get out of whack because the regulatory systems are impaired.

However, it takes a lot of abuse to hinder the regulators. Normal healthy people cause cholesterol deposits in their arteries or even raise the amount of cholesterol circulating in their bloodstream just by eating more cholesterol (provided other conditions such as total dietary calories and activity levels remain the same). Yet it is easy to raise blood cholesterol levels by stress, emotion, or even eating too many calories or too little vitamin C.

Some imbalances can be corrected by factors other than the primary factors involved, thanks to the complexities of the regulating mechanisms. As an example, too much carbohydrate in the diet can increase the triglyceride level of the blood. (Triglycerides are chemicals produced in the process of converting excess carbohydrates into stored body fat and are linked to heart disease.) The triglyceride level can be returned to an ideal range either by normalizing the dietary carbohydrate level or by increasing the L-carnitine content of the diet. (L-carnitine is an amino acid–like compound that helps control fat metabolism.)

Similarly, too much fat in the diet increases the amount of harmful peroxides in the body. Reducing the amount of fat in the diet will reduce the peroxide levels, but so will increasing the amount of vitamin E, selenium, and other antioxidant nutrients in the diet.

There are nutrients that normalize blood cholesterol levels and other nutrients that keep blood cells slippery and free from the type of clotting that causes heart attacks. Fatty foods tend to increase cholesterol levels and cause the blood cells to stick together. Lowering the fat content of the diet reduces the risk of heart disease by improving blood quality. Certain nutrients available in concentrated form as food supplements can maintain the ideal quality of blood even under adverse conditions.

These vital nutrients maintain normal cholesterol and triglyceride levels and proper cell slipperiness—even when excessive fats are consumed. The amounts of these nutrients that are required to achieve ideal blood quality depend on the overall diet and differ from person to person. However, the differences are slight, and convenient supplementation ranges will be discussed shortly.

Real Risk Factors

When one says that too much fat in the diet is a risk factor, what he or she is really saying is that excessive dietary fat causes chemical changes in the blood, blood cells, and arteries that result in heart disease. What is overlooked is that other dietary factors can also cause these changes in body chemistry. Similarly, still other dietary factors can prevent the changes associated with excessive fats from occurring.

The real risk factors are the intermediate chemicals produced that actually damage the blood cells or arteries. If we can reduce the levels of these chemical intermediates, then we can reduce heart disease. It really makes no difference how we reduce the chemical intermediates as long as we reduce them without harming the body. Yes, excessive fats can cause the damage via the intermediates, but if we focus only on the fats, then we neglect the other factors that can produce the same damage.

The "prudent" approach is to control the fats in the diet at about 20% to 30% of the total calorie content. The "alternative" approach is to control the real risk factors—the chemical intermediates.

Thus, it becomes important to identify the real risk factors. The real risk factors are not fats, dietary cholesterol, cigarettes, and lack of exercise, but are low-density lipoproteins (LDL), high blood-platelet adhesion index, triglycerides, benzo(a)pyrene (BP), and trace-element deficiencies.

Other Theories May Be Better

Cholesterol is getting all of the attention, but there is more to heart health than blood cholesterol levels. Evidence continues to grow showing that vitamin B-6 levels are related to heart disease incidence. Heart attacks may be higher when the vitamin B-6 levels are lower than a level that is higher than the Recommended Dietary Allowance.

Although the medical community focuses on cholesterol, it has long been known that about 20% of heart attack deaths have been due to coronary artery spasms, which are related not to deposits in the arteries, but to levels of the mineral magnesium and the amino acid tryptophan. Also, congestive heart failure is related to muscle tissue strength (cardiomyopathy), which is related to Coenzyme Q-10 (CoQ-10) and carnitine, not cholesterol. (CoQ-10 is a newly discovered nutrient that was discussed in Chapter 5 on slowing the aging process.)

There are other theories of heart disease that involve estrogen-related hormones and amino acids, not cholesterol or cholesterol carriers. The question is not whether these competing theories on heart disease are right or wrong; the question is how much heart disease is explained by these minority theories. Of the percentage of heart-disease deaths caused by clogged arteries, what percentage of these are caused by high levels of low-density lipoprotein-carried cholesterol, and what percentage are caused by low vitamin B-6 levels or high estradiol hormone levels?

A new, growing segment of the scientific community believes that heart disease develops in three stages: initiation, progression, and termination [Addis, P. B., *Food & Nutrition News* 62(2):7–11 (March/April 1990).

The initiation phase is caused by arterial injury due to free radicals, oxidative compounds, insulin, and/or high blood pressure. The progression phase causes plaque to build up by the action of foam cells, apolipoprotein, or low-density lipoprotein. The termination phase results in a myocardial infarction or arterial spasm due to sticky blood cells resulting from oxidative damage, pressure damage, or nutrient deficiencies.

Theories Not Involving Dietary Cholesterol or Fat

The major theories not involving either dietary cholesterol or fat are as follows:

- monoclonal proliferation
- arterial injury
- estradiol
- vitamin B-6 deficiency—homocysteine
- high blood insulin levels
- fibrinogen
- immune damage after viral infection
- genetics

Several scientists note that each of these theories has more scientific support than the popular dietary cholesterol theory. Each theory can explain the disease/no disease incidence on a clear-cut positive/negative basis, rather than disease/no disease being dependent on a component being elevated over a normal value.

Problems with Existing Studies and Data

Proponents and opponents criticize each other's results, often for the same reasons:

- insufficient numbers
- highly selected participants
- too short a time
- other parameters not eliminated

As an example, diet changes may produce short-term changes in blood values that disappear over a long time period. Or a study may be too short to demonstrate plaque formation or regression. Or inappropriate animal models may be used, such as vegetarian rabbits that must handle dietary cholesterol or rodents that manufacture their own vitamin C, which has an effect on blood cholesterol.

There may be inbred strains used that are not appropriate

to the heterogeneity of the human population. Or blood cholesterol may be measured in isolation instead of the total body cholesterol pool. If the blood cholesterol level changes, what accounts for the change? Less synthesis? Greater excretion? Less absorption? Migration into liver, muscle, or arteries?

Total blood cholesterol may be measured instead of cholesterol fractions. Or total calories may not be considered. Or other factors may be included without the effect of each being determined.

Or values may be termed "normal" that are really too high and not optimal. Cholesterol values near 300 mg/dl may be so far above ideal that not much difference would show with a 10% reduction.

Lack of Vitamin B-6 Causes Heart Disease

The evidence involving low vitamin B-6 levels and heart disease has been accumulating for years, and it is now time to pay more attention to vitamin B-6. Before discussing the new studies, let's review the background.

Vitamin B-6 is involved in hundreds of body processes. Proteins, carbohydrates, and fats are all processed in the body via enzymes that utilize vitamin B-6 as a cofactor. The regulation of cholesterol production in the body from food components absorbed in the ileum section of the intestine by vitamin B-6 has been known since 1950, and early vitamin B-6 heart disease research concentrated on fats and cholesterol.

In 1951 scientists learned that rhesus monkeys fed high-cholesterol diets developed humanlike arterial plaques when they were vitamin B-6-deficient, but not when they were well supplied with vitamin B-6. Even when the cholesterol level was four times higher in the high-vitamin-B-6-diet monkeys, they didn't develop the cholesterol plaques that the vitamin B-6-deficient monkeys did on their lower-cholesterol diets.

In 1956 these experiments with monkeys were confirmed, and experiments by other researchers using dogs and chickens produced the same results.

In 1962 scientists became curious about the high levels of

the amino acid homocysteine in the urine of two girls who died in their teens with extensive vascular disease and cholesterol plaques. The teenagers appeared as if they had the arteries of very old persons suffering from atherosclerosis.

Homocysteine is normally produced as the body processes proteins. Normally the body continues to process homocysteine into another amino acid called cystathionine. Cystathionine in turn is processed into other important compounds.

However, if there is not enough vitamin B-6 available, the body can't convert all of the homocysteine into cystathionine. As a result, homocysteine, a very toxic substance, circulates in the blood until it is excreted in the urine.

Figure 16.1

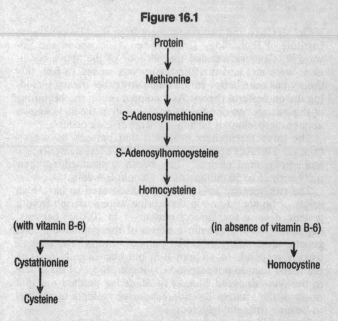

Vitamin B-6 is required to metabolize the food amino acid methionine into cysteine. Without eduaquate amounts of vitamin B-6, the intermediate metabolic amino acid, homocysteine, cannot be completely converted into cystathionine. As a result, homocysteine is converted into homocystine, which causes artery damage and heart disease.

In 1969 Dr. Kilmer McCully of Harvard University and the Massachusetts General Hospital tied the pieces together and presented a theory of heart disease for testing. If his theory was correct, he would have to show the following:

1. Animals develop atherosclerosis when homocysteine is injected into their bloodstream.
2. Vitamin B-6-deficient animals and humans have significantly more homocysteine in their urine than those receiving adequate vitamin B-6.
3. Atherosclerotic patients have low vitamin B-6 blood levels.
4. Atherosclerotic patients have high homocysteine blood levels.

Dr. McCully and two researchers from the Massachusetts Institute of Technology, Drs. Stephen A. Raymond and Edward R. Gruberg, verified that all four of the above conditions were met and that the theory was sound. In fact, this theory has been better verified than any other theory, including the cholesterol theory. As I pointed out in the beginning of this section, no one theory explains all of the facts known about atherosclerosis or how all heart disease occurs.

The three researchers proposed that persons having vitamin B-6 intakes above the RDA will have less heart disease and stroke than normal. They began supplementing their diets with 25 to 50 milligrams of vitamin B-6 daily.

The two teenage girls that were discovered to have high levels of homocysteine in their urine were suffering from a genetic disease that affects perhaps 1 in 100,000 persons, depending on the genetic makeup of the population. This genetic abnormality is called homocystinuria. The disease usually responds to vitamin B-6, but occasionally persons are found that do not respond to vitamin B-6. A 1983 article in the *New England Journal of Medicine* pointed out that many of the vitamin B-6 nonresponsive patients responded to betaine (trimethylglycine).

I would like to suggest that these patients may not have responded to vitamin B-6 because they could not form the active form of vitamin B-6, which is pyridoxal-5-phosphate (P-5-P or PLP). This "preformed" active vitamin B-6 is now available in supplements.

In 1984 Dr. E. J. Calabrese of the University of Massachusetts published an article in *Medical Hypothesis* that added more data to the theory. Diets often associated with heart disease, such as diets rich in meats and dairy products, are high in methionine, an amino acid that is directly converted to homocysteine by the body, and such diets do not provide adequate vitamin B-6 to compensate for the increased level of methionine.

More weight was added to the theory in 1985. Dr. W. J. Serfontein and colleagues at the University of Pretoria measured the P-5-P levels in men having had heart attacks within the preceding twenty-four hours and then compared those with the levels of healthy subjects. He found that the P-5-P levels of the heart-attack victims was slightly lower and the those of healthy persons. This is a highly significant difference.

In Dr. Serfontein's study he found that the cholesterol levels of the heart-attack victims was slightly lower and the HDL slightly higher. The researchers concluded that P-5-P level was a more sensitive indicator of heart-attack risk than total cholesterol or HDL cholesterol level. They also suggested that vitamin B-6 deficiency may influence the development of heart disease through the accumulation of homocysteine and/or some of its derivatives.

Dr. Serfontein's group expanded their P-5-P studies to smokers in 1986. It was discovered that the P-5-P levels of smokers averaged 9.2 nanograms per milliliter, whereas that of nonsmokers averaged 13.0. Again, this is a highly significant difference that can help explain the increased risk of heart disease among smokers, as well as establish another link of evidence for the vitamin B-6/homocysteine theory of heart disease. This could be added as point five to the four points suggested by Dr. McCully.

In 1987 folic acid deficiency was also associated with elevated homocysteine blood levels. Folic acid supplements were found to lower homocysteine levels quickly.

In 1989 the results of two studies were published by a Dutch group led by Drs. Frans Kok and Hans Valkenburg in the *American Journal of Cardiology*.[1] They studied eighty-four heart-attack patients and eighty-four healthy subjects and again confirmed that P-5-P levels of the blood plasma and red blood cells were lower in the heart-attack patients. The doctors suggest that "low levels of vitamin B-6 may increase the risk of heart attack."

At an international conference held in Philadelphia in 1989 researchers reported that a high percentage of persons above sixty-five years of age are deficient in vitamin B-6 and suggested that increased amounts taken throughout adulthood would reduce this deficient state.

The blossoming of this theory among scientists is witnessed by the coverage devoted to the theory in the conservative *Nutrition Reviews*.[2] *Nutrition Reviews* remarked, "It is possible that even in the general population, homocysteine might constitute a risk factor for the development of premature vascular disease, a hypothesis supported by the finding of an association between moderate homocysteinemia and cardiovascular disease in a number of studies."

Nutrition Reviews concludes, "In view of the importance of vascular disease and the relative safety of and low cost of folic acid, long-term controlled clinical trials would seem to be warranted both in patients with normal and in those with elevated plasma levels of homocysteine." Amen! But don't forget vitamin B-6!

I recommend that persons have their blood and urine tested for homocysteine to see if they are at risk, and if so, they should seek to reduce their homocysteine levels with vitamin B-6. If they are nonresponsive to vitamin B-6, then they should try P-5-P, betaine, and folic acid. An alternative is just to make sure we all have adequate folic acid and vitamin B-6 or P-5-P in our diets.

Arterial Wall Damage

Heart disease is usually the result of artery disease. Arteries that have cholesterol deposits are actually diseased arteries. And the "cholesterol deposits" are not simple deposits of cholesterol; the narrowings in the arteries are plaque material consisting of protein fibers, fats, carbohydrates, and cholesterol. The plaque material has not been deposited on the artery wall but has been formed in the middle layer of the artery and grown inward toward the lumen (opening) through which the blood flows.

This is the monoclonal proliferation theory of heart disease.[3] It is based on the fact that one mutated cell in the middle layer of the artery proliferates and grows wildly, mutated.

The plaque forms because the force of the flowing blood (especially when blood pressure is high) injures the artery lining, allowing chemicals in the blood, such as benzo(a)pyrene (BP) from cigarette smoke, to penetrate more easily and mutate artery muscle cells in the middle layer of the artery.

The antioxidant group of nutrients, especially vitamins A, C, and E, beta-carotene, Pycnogenol and the trace mineral selenium, protects the artery cells against the mutations that lead eventually to atherosclerosis (plaque in the arteries), and thence to a greater probability of blood blockage to the heart.

(An in-depth discussion by Drs. B. Hennig and C. K. Chow of the role of antioxidant nutrients in preventing endothelial cell injury by lipid peroxidation appears in *Free Radicals in Biology and Medicine*.[4])

A related theory is that cholesterol does not enter into artery deposits until it and/or its lipoprotein carriers are oxidized.

Sex Hormone

Another interesting theory that so far is almost perfectly supported by the evidence relates to the amount of the female sex hormone estradiol that is in the blood of men.

Dr. Gerald B. Phillips of New York City's St. Luke's-Roosevelt Hospital Center has found that the blood level of estradiol in men is a much better indicator of heart disease risk than cholesterol or HDL/LDL ratio.[5] Dr. Phillips and his colleagues have conducted two studies that are very informative, but ignored.

In their second study, which was published in 1983, sixty-one men who had heart attacks were compared to sixty-one men free of clinical evidence of heart disease. The men averaged seventy years of age, with a range from sixty-one to eighty-eight. The men were matched exactly with men of the same age and other risk factors. Among healthy men, blood levels of the female sex hormone were about thirty picograms per milliliter of blood. Among those with heart disease the estradiol levels were about thirty-seven picograms per milliliter.

In the study, blood samples were drawn from volunteers by physicians in Framingham, Massachusetts, frozen, and shipped to Dr. Phillips's laboratory in New York. The blood samples were identified only by number, and there was no way in which Dr. Phillips could have known which were from healthy volunteers and which were from those with heart disease.

Dr. Phillips analyzed the blood samples for many compounds, including cholesterol, estradiol, and the male sex hormone testosterone. Dr. Phillips mailed back his results to the Framingham physicians, along with his predictions of which were the healthy and which were the heart-attack victims. He was able to identify correctly nearly every one of the heart patients and the healthy persons by their estradiol levels alone. Testosterone levels did not vary significantly.

Of the fifteen men with the highest estradiol levels, thirteen had coronary heart disease. Of the fifteen men with the highest cholesterol levels, only three had had coronary heart disease.

Both heredity and diet can affect estradiol levels. Important nutrients that affect estradiol levels in men are vitamin B-6, magnesium, choline, inositol, and vitamin E. It is also possible that a heart attack could increase estradiol levels, so more research is needed here. Unfortunately, the great emphasis on cholesterol precludes grant money being awarded for this research.

Insulin

There is evidence that a long-term high blood level of insulin damages the arteries and causes the buildup of cholesterol deposits. Dr. Gerald M. Reaven of the Stanford University School of Medicine has studied insulin levels, resistance, and the incidence of heart disease. His summary publication in 1988 has attracted the attention of several researchers.[6]

If high insulin levels are related to heart disease, *then many of those who are steering away from fats and cholesterol are exposing themselves to greater risk from their high-carbohydrate diet.*

Dr. Reaven's conclusions are supported by an Italian group at Parma University headed by Dr. Ivana Zavaroni. They found that persons with high insulin levels also had higher blood pressure, lower HDL, and other risk factors.[7] The cause of the latter was high insulin—and not the other way around. The high insulin came first.

In France, a team headed by Dr. Annick Fontbonne at the French National Institute of Health and Medical Research confirmed this link in a fifteen-year study of 7,000 Paris policemen. The 169 policemen who died of heart disease had blood insulin levels averaging 20% higher than normal.

The researchers concluded, "Our studies indicate that the earliest marker of a higher coronary heart disease mortality is an elevation of blood insulin level."

It is important to distinguish cause from effect. When it rains we see a lot of umbrellas—but the umbrellas don't cause the rain. In fact, the rain doesn't "cause" the umbrellas. It can be safely said that rain is associated with umbrellas. The cause of umbrellas is people who don't want to get wet when they go into the rain.

The so-called link between blood cholesterol and heart disease may be that heart disease causes high blood cholesterol and not vice versa. At least in this case, it may turn out that high blood insulin causes the damage that leads to heart disease and also to high blood cholesterol.

There is evidence to show that a genetic factor that causes high blood pressure also causes high blood cholesterol. It is thought that in this case the heart disease is caused by the high blood pressure, not by the high blood cholesterol, which just happens to accompany the former.

The genetic link may also be involved in the high blood insulin level. The resistance of cells to taking up insulin from the blood may be genetically determined. And of course, there is a dietary link involving chromium and the glucose tolerance factor (GTF). GTF aids the cells in using insulin and thus helps keep insulin levels low. There is also a life-style link, as body fat increases insulin resistance and causes blood levels of insulin to increase.

Fibrinogen

The Framingham study that has led to most of the theories about cholesterol levels and heart disease risk has now produced some interesting facts about another risk factor, the blood level of a blood-clotting factor called fibrinogen. In a twelve-year follow-up of 1,300 persons whose blood levels of fibrinogen were measured in 1968, those who developed heart disease had fibrinogen levels in the upper two thirds of all the values.

The Framingham group included Drs. William Kannel, Phillip Wolf, William Castelli, and Ralph D'Agostino. These are prominent researchers, and the publication of their data in the *Journal of the American Medical Association* should also draw attention.[8] However, it seems that almost all available funds for research are tied up in cholesterol projects.

Problems with the Existing Cholesterol Research

Lately there has been more heat than light as the cholesterol proponents have decided that people would benefit if they put science behind and use—in good faith—Madison Avenue tactics.

MRFIT

One of the largest studies used to justify the use of diet and drugs to lower blood cholesterol levels was the Multiple Risk Factor Intervention Trial (MRFIT). Results of the MRFIT study were released in 1982 amid great fanfare by the National Heart, Lung and Blood Institute (NHLBI) of the National Institutes of Health. According to the agency and involved researchers, the data showed that a 1% reduction in blood cholesterol level results in a 2% drop in the risk of heart disease. You will see this figure used over and over as if it were true.

The published study proved nothing, as later admitted by the NHLBI. This is discussed later in this chapter. However, a later study—a ten-year follow-up of the people in the first study—indicates that they did receive a benefit from the total program, but no evidence was presented to show benefit from the dietary portion of the program.

The point is that two years after the first study was published a preemptive strike was made by the Lipid Research Clinic–Coronary Primary Prevention Trial (LRC-CPPT) without scientific justification. Before their claims were published for peer review, they held press conferences to announce that the debate was over—what little there was—and that they had conclusive proof that lowering dietary cholesterol and fat prevented heart disease.

The LRC-CPPT group told the media on January 12, 1984, that "in summary, the LRC-CPPT is the first study to demonstrate conclusively that the risk of coronary heart disease can be reduced by lowering blood cholesterol. For each 1% fall in cholesterol, a 2% reduction in heart attack risk can be expected. These results have widespread implications for many millions of Americans and, if applied, have the potential to markedly reduce the large number of heart attacks and heart attack deaths presently experienced in this country and elsewhere."

However, the conclusion in the *Journal of the American Medical Association*[9] is significantly more conservative. "The LRC-CPPT findings show that reducing total cholesterol by lowering LDL-cholesterol levels can diminish the incidence of CHD morbidity and mortality in men at high risk for CHD because of raised LDL-cholesterol levels. This clinical trial provides strong evidence for a causal role for these lipids in the pathogenesis of CHD."

Following this preemptive strike, the LRC group called for the National Heart, Blood and Lung Institute and the American Heart Association (AHA) to lead the way in directing large expenditures of government funds to educate the general public now that "conclusive proof" was finally at hand. All health professionals and their organizations were asked to increase this effort to inform the public of these findings.

The National High Cholesterol Education Program was proposed, and it was turned down at that time because it was deemed immature. However, the AHA went full steam ahead with what it felt was "smoking gun evidence."

More on this later!

The LRC-CPPT Study

According to the press briefing, the clinical trial addressed primary prevention of coronary heart disease. The group felt that a test of the hypothesis that a cholesterol-lowering diet by itself would reduce heart disease was not feasible because of (1) the large sample size that would be needed, (2) difficulties in conducting a double-blind study of diet, (3) the likelihood that other coronary heart disease risk factors would be changed in a non-blinded study, and (4) a cost that would exceed one billion dollars.

The LRC-CPPT study was an alternative approach to testing the cholesterol hypothesis. It used a potent cholesterol-lowering drug in participants with high blood LDL-cholesterol. Such an approach reduced the number of required study participants to a feasible level and allowed for a double-blind design.

The 3,806 men aged thirty-five to fifty-nine had blood cholesterol levels exceeding 265 mg/dl and had no clinical signs of CHD. It is estimated that 5% of men in this age group would have blood cholesterol levels this high. The period of observation ranged from seven to ten years.

Prior to trial initiation, men who did "not respond sufficiently to the diet (low in cholesterol) by the third or fourth visit were considered eligible for cholesterol-lowering by drugs, and therefore suitable for enrollment in the study." (This casts doubt on the suitability of the advice to reduce blood cholesterol with a low-cholesterol diet.)

Diet alone produced a 3.5% fall in total blood cholesterol and a 4% fall in LDL-cholesterol. After drug therapy total cholesterol fell 8.5% and LDL-cholesterol fell 12.6% from the diet-alone levels. This was less than anticipated, but it was discovered by packet count that not all participants took the recommended doses. The placebo group experienced 187 definite coronary heart disease deaths and/or definite non-fatal attacks, whereas the drug group experienced only 155 such definite events. This reflected a 24% reduction in definite coronary heart disease death and a 19% reduction in definite nonfatal heart attack. The greater the compliance to dose protocol, the greater the reduction in heart disease.

Those taking the full dose had a 25% reduction in blood cholesterol and a 50% reduction in CHD risk. This led to the "rough rule of thumb" that for each 1% fall in cholesterol there is a 2% fall in risk. This later became gospel in the news, and no mention was given about the effective range.

Other favorable differences in exercise electrocardiogram (ECG), angina, and bypass surgery were observed. However, the total deaths were about the same—seventy-one in the placebo group and sixty-eight in the drug group.

The drug cholestyramine caused minor side effects, such as constipation, heartburn, and other gastrointestinal problems. The potentiation of gastrointestinal carcinogens as discussed in the drug's warnings was noted by an increase in gastrointestinal cancers, but other cancers were decreased to yield comparable cancer incidences.

The major finding announced was that the LRC-CPPT study was the first study in humans to establish conclusively that lowering blood cholesterol reduces heart attacks and heart-attack deaths.

LRC-CPPT Criticism

An editorial in the *New England Journal of Medicine* said that the LRC-CPPT study had been wrongly interpreted to magnify the effect of the cholesterol-lowering drugs, and that these interpretations were further distorted by drug company advertising that "stretches the truth to the limits."[10,11]

The editorial discussed two studies of drug therapy for lowering high blood cholesterol levels, the LRC-CPPT and the Helsinki study. They produced similar results, and both were interpreted to show that the drugs significantly reduced incidence of heart disease.

Although the absolute difference in heart disease death rate between those taking the drugs and those not taking drugs was small, reports and advertising sought to claim otherwise. The absolute difference in fatal heart attacks in the LRC-CPPT between the two groups (drug and nondrug) was 1.7% (9.8% vs. 8.1%); it was reported as a 19% reduction. The Helsinki result of a 1.4% difference was presented as a 34% heart-attack-death reduction.

The editorial asked the question, "How does one weigh a benefit for fourteen people (Helsinki data) against the effects of treating 986 people who are not destined to benefit?"

The editorial pointed out that there were significant side effects and that other forms of premature death from the drugs could not be dismissed. In addition, depending on the drug, costs could be $700 to $1,500 a year. A sixty-year drug usage could cost as much as $90,000. Later we will examine a plan to treat twenty-five million Americans with drugs. A nice bit of business!

Considerable criticism of the claims made to the public followed the published results. Generally, the comments suggested that too much had been made of too little—that the results were being overinterpreted. The comments included:

(1) Very little can be concluded about diet, since there was no group not on a "cholesterol-lowering" diet. Diet was not a variable in the study.

(2) Very little can be concluded about diet, since the agent lowering the blood cholesterol level was a drug that could have produced its beneficial actions through mechanisms other than blood-cholesterol lowering. The effect of increasing or decreasing dietary cholesterol and/or fat was not studied.

(3) Overall mortality was not reduced.

(4) The results apply to middle-aged men with cholesterol levels above 265 mg/dl, and, as suggested in *Nature*,[12] reducing blood cholesterol from lower initial levels is of questionable benefit.

(5) The researchers did not make certain that the patients they reported to have died of coronary heart disease actually did succumb to that affliction. A recent study showed that only 53% of antemortem diagnoses matched postmortem findings.

(6) The "blinding" of participating subjects and the in-

vestigators was maintained in less than 50% of the cases for over seven years, and the research group was biased.

(7) As mentioned earlier, rather than a 19% decrease in mortality, others see only a 1.5% difference (6.8 vs. 8.3) in 3,806 men. The actual percentage reduction was 0.43%. Critics see the incidence of CHD among treated patients as high, and the small difference in CHD experience over 7.4 years as evidence that cholestyramine is not a very effective drug (two men per year in every 10,000 on the drug). Cholestyramine has been on the market for seventeen years without arousing excitement among practicing physicians. How did the mortality of the placebo group compare to the expected mortality if the participants were not given a placebo or drug?

(8) Of eight clinics in the trial, four showed no difference, and one showed the opposite effect.

(9) The effect of blood-cholesterol lowering on impulsive homicidal and suicidal behavior was dismissed. But Dr. Virkkunen argues that there is a relationship in the *Journal of the American Medical Association*.[13] In nearly every clinical trial, the treated group did reduce its death rate from heart disease, but the members of the group died of something else—frequently cancer.[14] There is evidence to suggest that the drug or the drop in blood cholesterol may disturb alcohol metabolism or balance in those experiencing violent behavior and death. Perhaps cholesterol lowering is not always entirely safe for everyone.

(10) Gastrointestinal cancer increased by 700%.

(11) The results claimed to show a reduced number of nonfatal heart attacks, but the data were not statistically significant.[15,16]

(12) There is no evidence to support the assumption that dietary cholesterol has a "linear" effect on blood cholesterol for values below 265 mg/dl, which includes 95% of the population.

(13) There are more effective dietary measures to lower blood cholesterol than either restricting dietary cholesterol or using cholestyramine.

These strong criticisms by themselves, however, do not invalidate the truth of the hypothesis any more than the data validate a possible truth.

The Cholesterol Education Caper

So victory is claimed even though the science isn't there. You may ask what harm there is. The advice doesn't seem to cause any problems. The problem is that if they are wrong, people's efforts are misdirected. And giving up some nourishing foods can lower health unless care is taken to keep the nutrient level of the altered diet high. And there is the stress of avoiding popular foods. But just because the studies are poor, that doesn't mean the answer is wrong.

The fact that the great National Cholesterol Education Program is a gigantic money-maker for the supporters has not been overlooked. The screening programs bring in more customers to the physicians for treatment; they buy more expensive drugs; the testing laboratories have more customers; and everybody is happy. That is, they are happy until they find their blood cholesterol levels don't change for very long.

The admitted goal of the National Cholesterol Education Program is to place 25 million Americans on lifelong drug treatment for high cholesterol. According to *Nutrition Week,*[17] Judy Wagner of the U.S. Office of Technology Assessment has said that the bill for cholesterol testing will be $22 million a year. It will cost billions more each year for dietary advice, physician services, and a lifelong drug habit, mostly paid by individual patients.

Nutrition Week went on to point out,

The campaign is an expensive fraud. . . . The heart icons have known from the start these facts:

1. No relationship could be established between dietary cholesterol and blood cholesterol.
2. The cholesterol drug habit must begin at an early age and continue for a lifetime to have any effect. Yet, after an expenditure of $100,000 or more, the user at best could expect to live an additional three to six months. After age fifty, the period when most heart attacks occur, no relationship can be shown between blood cholesterol level and coronary heart disease.

"Know your cholesterol number," we are told. Which number? The meaning of your blood cholesterol number depends on the test used to measure it. I am not referring to the quick tests done at malls and in doctors' offices, but the tests done in hospital or clinic laboratories.

The "official" guidelines are based on the LRC method, but most laboratories use the SMAC or ACA methods. Table 16.1 compares the cholesterol numbers obtained by the three different methods. Always ask your doctor which method was used and what are the normal and high ranges for that test procedure.

The cholesterol testing is ludicrous. People are stopping at "health fairs" in shopping centers to have their blood cholesterol checked. The lack of fasting, the untrained operators, the uncalibrated instruments, the improper blood extraction methods, etc. finally led the FDA to speak out. It isn't that the equipment *can't* be operated correctly—it's that the equipment *isn't* operated properly, and the blood samples aren't correctly drawn.

Dr. Richard Kusserow, inspector general of the Department of Health and Human Services, sent out press releases stating that "many public cholesterol screenings are inaccurate, unsanitary, and improperly conducted."

The tests may seem cheap, but not when you are sent to a physician for treatment you don't need or have the test repeated by a proper laboratory procedure.

TABLE 16.1
Comparison of Cholesterol Test Procedure Numbers

MODERATE RISK

Age	LRC method	SMAC method	ACA method
20–29	200	225	240
30–39	220	250	265
40 +	240	275	290

HIGH RISK

20–29	220	250	265
30–39	240	275	290
40 +	260	295	315

Near the end of 1989 criticism was taking its toll on the program and NHLBI. *Nutrition Week*[18] reported that NHLBI believed that "it may have made a mistake in assuming that the relationship between (blood) cholesterol and coronary heart disease can be extrapolated from data gathered on white middle-aged males. The institute acknowledges that it has no clinical data to support recommendations to lower (blood) cholesterol levels in women or in elderly men."

As mentioned earlier by *Nutrition Week*, some wonder about the concern about cholesterol in men under fifty years of age when only 7% of fatal heart attacks occur before age fifty-five. Above fifty years of age cholesterol levels do not seem to correlate with heart disease incidence or heart disease death.

The Surgeon General at that time, Dr. C. Everett Koop, was about to retire and freely offered his personal view: "I think the cholesterol bubble is about to burst." Earlier he had stated that the National Cholesterol Education Program lacked sufficient justification, according to *Nutrition Week*.[19]

The criticism came at a time when the NHLBI was about to formally introduce its official low-fat diet recommendations. The NHLBI announced that the recommendations would be delayed until February 1990 "for further review."

In mid-December, 1989, the U.S. Congress opened a public hearing into the matter. In spite of Congressional shock, the National Cholesterol Education Program continued without abatement. U.S. Representative Ron Wyden of Oregon said the program "defies common sense and is contrary to public interest."

The American Heart Association Prostitutes Itself

As the National Cholesterol Education Program got underway others saw how they, too, could make money. The American Heart Association devised a gimmick. The AHA would sell its endorsement to manufacturers. For a stiff fee a manufacturer could buy an AHA seal of approval, called "Heart-Guide," for its labels. The HeartGuide designated a product as being heart-safe, at least in the eyes of the AHA. It's bad enough to see "no cholesterol" potato chips. (Only animal products have cholesterol.) Will there be "no cholesterol" cigarettes? Well, we don't have to worry about what strange products the HeartGuide will be on, because it was banned by the U.S. government.

In October 1989 Lester Crawford, administrator of the Food Safety and Inspection Service of the U.S. Department of Agriculture, labeled the HeartGuide as misleading and not supported by adequate scientific justification. He also pointed out "attempts to label foods as 'good' or 'bad' using *inadequate* nutritional criteria . . . will undermine the public confidence in the science of nutrition and the scientific community."

According to the October 26, 1989 *Nutrition Week*, Richard Sullivan, executive vice president of the Association of Food Industries, described the HeartGuide program as "an extortion racket." He was referring to the price that AHA would charge to evaluate food products as candidates for AHA endorsement. Depending on the market share held by a particular food product, "AHA said it will charge over a million dollars per product."

The HeartGuide contracts would have been in effect for a minimum of three years, so it would have been a three-million-dollar investment. Of course, the consumer would have ended up paying for the fee as an advertising cost.

Just how much would it have cost the AHA to read a label, verify the analysis, and determine if a product met its guidelines? Why wouldn't that remain valid until a formula was changed?

Their extortionary approach reminds me of the old joke in which a boss asks his new secretary if she would make love to him for a million dollars. She replied, "For a million dollars I'd do just about anything." The boss inquired, "Would you do it for fifty dollars?" Indignantly she said, "Just what do you take me for, a prostitute?" He grinned. "We have already established what you are; we are just haggling over the price."

May the HeartGuide rest in peace, and may the AHA use its money to conduct research into the other aspects of heart disease.

The Debate Is Renewed

Thus, in spite of claims of victory by the low-cholesterol proponents, the debate continues. After thousands of animal studies and dozens of major epidemiological studies, no clinical study has conclusively shown that dietary cholesterol and/or fat causes heart disease.

Major studies have included the WHO Coronary Prevention Study, the Coronary Clubs, the Pooling Project Research Group Study, the Chicago Gas Project, the Western Electric Study, the North Karelia–Kupio Study, the Los Angeles VA Hospital Project, the London Medical Research Council Low-Fat Diet Study, MRFIT, the Oslo Study, the Tecumseh Trial, etc., etc., etc.

However, the LRC-CPPT study has shifted the focus of the debate. There is less dissent over the merit of lowering blood cholesterol in highly elevated blood cholesterol individuals. Most of the dissent is aimed at recommendations that blood cholesterol be lowered in the population as a whole and in the effect of dietary cholesterol on blood cholesterol in typical healthy persons.

The debate was brought to the public's attention in September 1989 by an article in the *Atlantic Monthly* by Thomas Moore. The cover headline was "The Cholesterol Myth." This was followed with the shocker to the general public, "Lowering your cholesterol is next to impossible with diet, and often dangerous with drugs—and it won't make you live any longer."

The article claimed that and then detailed "how the NHLBI, AHA and AMA ignored [that] the results of the most expensive research effort yet mounted failed to substantiate long held beliefs that cholesterol causes coronary heart disease. Instead, those icons of medical research chose to whip the American people into a cholesterol hysteria to promote nutritional practices that have yet to demonstrate the saving of a single life from lowering cholesterol."

Points made in the article included:

(1) "The government's $115-million, seven-year-long clinical trials with more than 12,000 participants proved that following a strict diet does not lower cholesterol levels

enough to have an effect on deaths from coronary heart disease."

(That's because they focus on fats and cholesterol. In the next chapter I will show you how to lower cholesterol thirty points in thirty days using vitamins, minerals, and other supplements.)

(2) "The public health campaign against cholesterol was created by a coalition that had developed too big a stake in the cholesterol theory to face up to the increasingly apparent failure of experiments to confirm it. The coalition included a small but powerful group of cholesterol researchers in key medical schools who conducted the major experiments, and officials of NHLBI, which for ten years had committed more than half its clinical trials budget to cholesterol research.

"When the NHLBI's biggest cholesterol-lowering trial failed to produce the predicted results, it claimed success anyway and began the cholesterol campaign. It was joined by drug companies with millions invested in developing cholesterol-lowering drugs. The campaign was eagerly embraced by the American Medical Association, which told its members about the large number of additional laboratory tests and office visits that a campaign against cholesterol program might create.

"Together the agencies and companies ignored the growing chorus of criticism in the medical community and scientific journals. For example, since plans for a national cholesterol campaign were first announced in 1985, critical articles or editorials appeared in the *Annals of Internal Medicine, Circulation, The Mayo Clinic Proceedings, Medical Care,* the *Journal of the American College of Cardiology,* and the *Journal of the American Medical Association.*

"Strategists at NHLBI also discovered that while the public was highly sensitized to the cholesterol question, a majority of doctors weren't convinced that diet was important in preventing coronary heart disease. It funded a special research project to learn how most effectively to change physicians' minds on the diet question."

Fabrication and Admitted Errors

After the public embarrassment caused by the *Atlantic Monthly* article the National Heart, Lung and Blood Institute (NHLBI) admitted that the key heart study used to justify the massive cholesterol intervention campaign was flawed from the outset.

Dr. Basil Rifkind, chief of the institute's Lipid Metabolism and Atherogenesis Branch, admitted in November 1989 that the MRFIT study was badly designed. Dr. Rifkind acknowledged that the experimental and control groups received the same basic treatment. Therefore, the data could lead to findings that neither the drugs nor diets significantly lowered the risk of death for individuals treated for high blood cholesterol levels.

Nutrition Week,[20] published by the Community Nutrition Institute, pointed out that Dr. Rifkind's acknowledgment raised more questions than it answered.

"If the study design was flawed, why was so obvious of a fault so easily overlooked, particularly since MRFIT was the largest and most expensive cholesterol study to be funded by the NHLBI, a study described by the agency as providing the final answer to the cholesterol question? Why has NHLBI waited so long to suggest it made such an error? Why has NHLBI chosen to disown MRFIT only when the public is becoming aware that its data threaten the credibility of the cholesterol program? Until these questions are answered, the Rifkind statement can be viewed as an effort by NHLBI to jettison the MRFIT data while claiming the cholesterol program is justified on the basis of other studies."

Two years ago a key investigator long associated with the cholesterol study was found to have fabricated his research results.[21]

Major Cholesterol/Fat Theories

The major dietary emphasis has changed from a low-cholesterol, high–polyunsaturated fat diet to a low-cholesterol, low-fat diet through the years.

There have been many research groups involved. Excellent reviews of the literature can be obtained by searching under any of the following names: E. Ahrens, Jr.; M. Altshule; W. Castelli; M. DeBakey; A. Harper; W. Kannel; A. Keys; D. Kritchevsky; R. Levy; G. Mann; M. Oliver; R. Olson; K. Oster; E. Pinckney; R. Reiser; B. Rifkind; and J. Stamler.

The researchers offer various hypotheses on diet and blood cholesterol. The main research lines are as follows:

- low dietary cholesterol intake lowers blood cholesterol
- low dietary cholesterol and high dietary polyunsaturated fat intake lowers blood cholesterol
- low dietary cholesterol and high polyunsaturated-to-saturated fat ratio lowers blood cholesterol
- low dietary cholesterol and low fat intake lowers blood cholesterol
- increasing other nutrients lowers blood cholesterol
- decreasing other dietary components such as caffeine lowers blood cholesterol
- blood cholesterol varies with total calories
- no dietary factors significantly affect blood cholesterol

There are other variations on the theme, and there are other themes as well. It is important to note that some scientists have epidemiological data to suggest that eating more cholesterol and saturated fats increases heart disease—even though the diet does not increase blood cholesterol levels or LDL.

There you have it! Every variation imaginable. Which is right? Are most of them right? There is still a lot to learn. You can follow them all, or you can pick and choose. The choice is yours. Time will tell who is correct. Don't take chances. Hedge your bet. Or in terms of cholesterol, don't put all of your eggs in one basket. Be prudent and be well-nourished, too.

Don't forget that moderate exercise is important, and personal stress may be a risk factor. Stress is not to be confused with hard work. Stress is doing what you are forced to do and don't enjoy.

Chapter 17 will show you how to lower your cholesterol by 30 points in 30 days.

17

Lowering Cholesterol
30 Points in 30 Days

———————————————————————————————

Blood cholesterol levels are usually kept in a normal range by a complex regulatory mechanism. When the diet is changed the regulatory mechanism adapts to this change and keeps the blood cholesterol normal. However, when the diet is deficient in the nutrients that keep the cholesterol regulatory mechanism working the blood cholesterol can become elevated. So it's not what you eat that raises blood cholesterol most, it's what you don't eat.

This chapter will discuss the nutrients that are most effective in keeping blood cholesterol normal. You may be pleased to know that it is easier, faster, and more effective to lower cholesterol with these nutrients than by making radical changes in your diet.

This chapter will also discuss the meaning of the cholesterol numbers and their recommended ranges. To better understand cholesterol, how it's regulated in the blood, and how certain nutrients influence blood cholesterol level, let's look at each of these factors.

Lipoprotein

Everyone "knows" that eating cholesterol increases the level of cholesterol in the blood and that that is what causes heart disease. In spite of that simple "fact" being repeated over and over again for more than fifty years, it doesn't seem to be true for the average person.

Only a relatively few individuals respond to increased dietary cholesterol with increased blood levels of cholesterol. (For the skeptics, a listing of modern studies that verify this point is given at the end of this chapter, references 1–13.) Body chemistry is just not that simple. There are several systems in the body that keep the amount of cholesterol circulating in the body within a fairly narrow range for each person.

Unless a genetically normal person upsets his regulatory mechanism by being deficient in certain vitamins and minerals or overstresses the body, his blood cholesterol level will not be affected by practical variations in dietary cholesterol.

Cholesterol is needed in the body to produce many other chemicals, ranging from sex hormones and bile to vitamin D and components of the immune system. These other chemicals are far too important for the body to rely solely on the diet to provide the needed cholesterol.

Vegetables contain no cholesterol; thus vegetarians would not survive if their bodies did not manufacture adequate cholesterol. Our bodies manufacture more cholesterol if we don't get enough in the diet. And when we eat more cholesterol than normal, our bodies merely adjust by cutting back on our own production. If still more massive amounts of cholesterol are eaten, then our bodies reduce the amount of cholesterol absorbed from the diet and increase cholesterol excretion.

The body has several control systems for cholesterol. If the blood level of cholesterol falls below a certain point, the liver compensates by manufacturing more; if the cholesterol blood levels rise above a certain level, then additional cholesterol is converted into bile and soon excreted.

These regulatory systems work well in the genetically normal, well-nourished, active individual. However, if you are deficient in vitamin C and are not very active, you can expect your regulatory mechanisms to be a little sluggish and imperfect. A "prudent" life-style helps maintain your regulatory systems by reducing the amount of compensation required by your body chemistry, but it can't compensate when the necessary nutrients are lacking.

There are other and easier ways of controlling the amount of cholesterol in your blood, but that is still focusing on the wrong event. The total amount of cholesterol in your blood is an irrelevant factor! That measurement is as useful in predicting heart disease as hat size or bra size. Have you noticed that most heart disease patients have normal cholesterol levels? And have you ever wondered why cholesterol deposits only occur in arteries—never in veins—although they both carry the same blood?

Cholesterol is not soluble in blood. Cholesterol is soluble in oil or fat. That's why cholesterol is found in animal fat. Unfortunately, this association with fat—and fat does affect blood cholesterol level to an extent—has resulted in many researchers associating changes in blood chemistry with the cholesterol rather than the fat.

Blood is a water-based mixture of various cells, simple chemicals, and special proteins that carry complex or water-insoluble chemicals. Cholesterol is needed by many organs in the body; it must be transported to these organs in the blood. Since cholesterol is insoluble in watery fluids, the body must supply a vehicle to carry the cholesterol. This is accomplished with a protein called lipoprotein.

Lipoproteins are similar to soaps. Soap dissolves oils and greases from skin and clothes and carries them away in the wash water. Yet oils and grease are insoluble in water. Soaps accomplish their task because one end of a soap molecule can dissolve oils and the other end is soluble in water. The same is true of lipoproteins. "Lipo" means "fat" to the chemist, so a lipoprotein molecule is part fat and part protein. The fat part of the lipoprotein is compatible with cholesterol, and the protein part is compatible with blood.

Lipoproteins consist of particles, each of which is a globule of lipid molecules surrounded by an apoprotein shell. "Apo" means "without or from." An apoprotein is the protein portion of a lipoprotein without the lipid portion. As a result, cholesterol, which by itself is not compatible with blood, can be carried in the bloodstream as a component of blood.

In fact, the body goes one step further. There are several lipoproteins. Cholesterol intended for different purposes is carried by different lipoproteins. When we ship the same item for different purposes, we often use different carriers. When manufacturers ship merchandise to retail stores for sale they use normal delivery trucks. When the consumers are finished with these items they are not sent back to the manufacturer by delivery truck but instead are sent to the dump in garbage trucks.

This, in essence, is what the body does. Cholesterol being removed from the bloodstream is carried by a special type of lipoprotein called high-density lipoprotein or HDL for short. This cholesterol is said to be "good" cholesterol in terms of heart disease and is returned to the liver for reprocessing or conversion to other compounds as part of a regulatory mechanism.

Other cholesterol is added to the bloodstream for easy assimilation by various organs (and, unfortunately, by arterial walls) and this cholesterol is carried by another type of lipoprotein called low-density lipoprotein or LDL for short. This cholesterol is said to be "bad" cholesterol in terms of heart disease.

Thus HDL is a "good guy," and LDL is a "bad guy." Evidence developed over the last ten years indicates that HDL is indeed protective against heart disease, and that LDL is a definite risk factor in heart disease. In fact, the most accurate indicator of heart disease risk is the level of LDL (and more specifically, lipoprotein(a) [Lp(a)]. Lp(a) consists of linked molecules of the protein portion of LDL called apolipoprotein(a) and LDL. LP(a) can transport cholesterol and deposit it in areas of the body where artery damage has occurred and it can interfere with the dissolution of clots in the bloodstream.

Perhaps you can see this more clearly if you think in terms of the trucks used in the earlier example. Think of LDL as being delivery trucks and HDL as being garbage trucks. It doesn't make any difference how many trucks you have as long as you have more "garbage" trucks than "delivery" trucks. Likewise, it's not so important as to how much cholesterol is in your blood, but as to how much bad cholesterol is in your blood. In medical terms, your total cholesterol level is not as important as either your LDL level or your LDL/ HDL ratio.

HDLs are actually particles containing about 50 percent fat and 50% apolipoproteins by weight. The fats are mostly phospholipids, cholesterol and triglycerides. The apolipoproteins are about 65% apolipoprotein A-I and about 30 percent apolipoprotein A-II. As later studies have shown, though physicians haven't put it into practice yet, apolipoprotein A-I is a better marker of heart disease risk than even HDL.

Since LDL is the bad guy, why should we worry about cholesterol and totally ignore LDL? The "alternative" strategy will concentrate on those factors known to decrease LDL and increase HDL.

Even more important, but not yet into the mainstream practice of cardiology, is that lipoprotein(a) should be monitored as the main indicator for heart disease risk. Drs. Matthias Rath and Linus Pauling have noted that this "bad" lipoprotein that is a reliable indicator or risk is related to the amount of vitamin C in the diet. When vitamin C blood levels are adequate, then Lp(a) levels are normal. [Proc. Natl. Acad. Sci., 87:6204-7 (August 1990)]

Drs. Rath and Pauling also note that vitamin C levels are low in heart patients and smokers. They also note that vitamin C levels are lower in arterial plaques than in other cells. Lp(a) above 30 milligrams per deciliter (mg/dl) doubles the risk of heart disease, and if the LDL is also elevated, the risk of heart disease is five times higher than normal.

Drs. Rath and Pauling believe that vitamin C deficiency not only increases the amount of Lp(a), but also allows more Lp(a) to penetrate the artery walls.

Free Radicals Help LDL Damage Arteries

Studies by Dr. Alex Sevanian of the University of Southern California indicate that free radicals can attack LDL and change its form so that LDL penetrates arteries more easily and leads to the accumulation of fat- and cholesterol-filled cells in the arteries. Antioxidant nutrients will protect against this damage.

Dr. Hermann Esterbauer of the University of Ganz, Austria found that LDL that becomes oxidized is attacked by the macrophages of the immune system. The macrophages are unable to digest the LDL particles and "die." The fat-filled "dead" macrophages accumulate and injure the arterial lining, resulting in plaque.

Researchers led by Dr. J. C. Fruchart of the Pasteur Institute in Lille, France gave volunteers with high LDL-cholesterol 1,000 IU of vitamin E daily for two months and found that they produced fewer "dead" fat-filled macrophages and had lower blood cholesterol.

Actually, a study published in *Acta Cardiologica* [44(6) (1989)] concludes that neither blood nor plasma cholesterol levels were reliable predictors of heart disease, but that having low levels of vitamin E was certainly a risk. This supports the hypothesis that vitamin E prevents atherosclerosis through the inhibition of oxidative lipoprotein modification.

A study at the University of Kentucky by Dr. B. Hennig showed that when artery tissues were well nourished with vitamin E they were protected against injury. However, when they were vitamin E deficient, oxidative stress caused many deleterious changes in the arteries. [*Internat. J. Vit. Nutr. Res.* 59: 273–279 (1989)]

In addition to vitamin E, the antioxidant nutrients vitamin C, beta-carotene, Pycnogenol and selenium have all been shown to reduce disease.

Before we look at reducing blood cholesterol levels or improving HDL/LDL ratios, let's look at the "official" guidelines for blood cholesterol levels and the "official" guidelines for eating cholesterol.

Consensus Guidelines on Serum Cholesterol

On December 13, 1985, a National Institutes of Health Consensus Development Conference on Lowering Blood Cholesterol to Prevent Heart Disease made five major recommendations. Three dealt with high-risk adults with serum cholesterol over 240 mg/dl who require identification and treatment; one dealt with a blanket recommendation that all Americans age two to ninety adopt low-cholesterol, fat-modified diets.

Even though voting has nothing to do with science, it should be noted that ten of the twenty-four speakers chosen for their anti-cholesterol leanings did not agree with universal diet modification.

The panel set as desirable cholesterol goals blood cholesterol levels less than 180 mg/dl for adults in their twenties, less than 200 mg/dl for those in their thirties, and less than 215 for those above forty. They urged aggressive treatment for those whose blood cholesterol levels are 40 mg/dl above those recommended levels.

A survey of thirty-one hospitals in Nebraska showed that norms for serum cholesterol were disparate from ideal values. In sixteen labs normative upper limits were 300 mg/dl. The study authors suggest 120–200 mg/dl as ideal.

The American Heart Association published its recommendation in 1982. The AHA established high blood cholesterol levels at higher values as shown in Table 17.1.

Table 17.2 lists the theoretical relative risks of various cholesterol levels compared to the suggested ideal of 180.

In 1985 a panel of "experts" convened at the National Heart, Lung and Blood Institute and published the guidelines

TABLE 17.1
1982 High Cholesterol Levels

Age	High Cholesterol	Normal	(Range)
20–24	212	180	(120–240)
25–29	234	180	(120–240)
30–34	258	205	(140–270)
35–39	267	205	(140–270)
40–44	260	225	(150–310)
45–49	275	225	(150–310)
50–54	274	245	(140–330)
55–59	280	245	(140–330)
60–64	287	. . . . . .	. . . .

presented in Table 17.3. They are nice, easy, symmetrical round numbers. Facts aren't always so convenient.

The AHA made the following dietary recommendations:

Phase I, for all Americans:
  Consume only 30% of your calories from fat; eat less than 300 mg cholesterol per day.

Phase II, for those having high blood cholesterol not controlled by Phase I:
  Consume lesss than 25% of calories as fat and less than 200–250 mg cholesterol per day.

Phase III, for those having high blood cholesterol not controlled by Phase II:
  Reduce calories from fat to 20% and keep cholesterol to 100–150 mg per day.

TABLE 17.2
Risks Relative to 180 Cholesterol

Cholesterol (mg/dl)	Risk of Heart Disease (compared to 180)
180–200	25% higher
200–220	200% higher
220–240	250% higher
240–260	300% higher
260–300	400% higher
>300	500% + higher

TABLE 17.3
1985 Cholesterol Goals

Age	Desired limit	Moderate risk	High risk
20–29	180	220	240
30–39	200	240	260
40+	220	260	280

There is nothing wrong with these guidelines *provided that the overall diet contains optimal amounts of vitamins and minerals.* In fact, such diets, including vegetarian diets, can indeed be very healthy. But don't concentrate on these factors and ignore other important factors such as total nourishment.

Reasonable advice would be not to remove good foods from the diet just because they have cholesterol in them. Do not add vegetable oils to the diet to change the ratio of polyunsaturates to saturates. Instead, lower total fats to less than 30% of the diet calories. Replace some saturated fats and vegetable oils (omega-two fats) with fish oils (omega-three fats) and gamma-linolenic acid—GLA—(omega-one fats) to balance the total fat complex of saturated fat, omega-one fat, omega-two fat, and omega-three fat.

Reduce dietary cholesterol only when the cholesterol is in high-calorie, low-nutrient food or when both of the following apply:

1. you have high blood cholesterol, and
2. your blood cholesterol decreases as you decrease dietary cholesterol.

Let's consider something much more important than total blood cholesterol level—the HDL level and the ratio of HDL to LDL.

Good HDL Levels

Regardless of the total cholesterol level, the HDL should be as high as possible. This relationship can be seen in Table 17.4. In a twelve-year follow-up study as part of the Framingham study, it was found that persons in the top 20% of HDL levels had only half the incidence of heart disease of those in the lowest 20%.[14]

However, don't get too excited about these figures until you examine Table 17.5 in the next section.

Factors that tend to improve HDL cholesterol levels are: reducing body fat; exercise; vitamins B-3, C, and E; chromium; fish oil; monounsaturated fats; and garlic and onions.

TABLE 17.4
HDL Levels and Risk of Heart Disease

HDL-cholesterol (mg/dl)	Coronary Heart Disease (per 1,000 men)
<25	170
25–44	100
45–64	60
65–74	40

Factors that tend to lower HDL cholesterol levels are: smoking; calories as sugar; and increased body fat.

The Total Cholesterol-to-LDL Ratio

Several studies have shown that the HDL-to-LDL ratio and its more popular variation, the total-cholesterol-to-HDL ratio (TC/HDL), are much better predictors of heart disease incidence than total blood cholesterol level alone.

Table 17.5 gives some comparisons from the Framingham study. Heart disease risk increases with increasing values of total cholesterol divided by HDL.

The Framingham researchers believe that the levels should be at least a 45 HDL, LDL under 130, and triglycerides

TABLE 17.5
Relative Risk by Total-Cholesterol-to-HDL Ratio

	Total Cholesterol	HDL	TC/HDL Ratio
Vegetarians	123	44	2.8
Marathoners	184	54	3.4
Goal	198	45	4.4
Average risk	260	45	5.8
Twice average risk	290	30	9.6
Thrice average risk	. . .	. .	24.0

under 150. They believe anything over a ratio of total cholesterol to HDL of 4.4 puts a person at risk. This is based on a total cholesterol of 200 and an HDL of 45.

What may be the best conventional cholesterol indicator developed so far has been developed by Dr. William E. Freeman, Jr. from the Bowling Green Study. Dr. Freeman uses a measurement that includes a cholesterol retention fraction figure that is defined as LDL minus HDL. His formula is as follows:

$$\text{Risk} = (\text{LDL} - \text{HDL})/\text{LDL}$$

As mentioned much earlier in this chapter in the lipoprotein section, the best markers of heart disease risk may be the apolipoproteins (apo's) that make up the HDL and LDL particles. In 1983 the *New England Journal of Medicine* article by Dr. James Maciejko and colleagues showed that apolipoprotein A-I was a better indicator of heart disease than HDL. Measuring your "apo" is 2.5 times more accurate than measuring LDL and twice as accurate as measuring HDL levels or the TC/HDL ratio.[15]

Improving TC/HDL and HDL/LDL Ratios

Several nutrients dramatically improve the TC/HDL ratio. Vitamin C, lecithin, and the chromium-containing glucose tolerance factor (GTF) all are extremely effective, and vitamin E also seems to be very effective according to some studies. All of the above nutrients are available as food supplements from most health food and drug stores. You can get them in a natural diet if you wish, but it's hard to measure how much you are getting. Have you seen extensive food tables for chromium? Try eating plenty of citrus fruits for vitamin C, eggs and soybeans for lecithin, and yeast for chromium-GTF.

Beta-Carotene

Preventing the oxidation of LDL and protecting the artery linings with antioxidants are more important than how much cholesterol is in the blood! More evidence of this was learned from the Harvard Physicians' Health Study. The antioxidant beta-carotene, which is the precursor of vitamin A, *cut heart disease and stroke incidence in half.*

Dr. J. Michael Gaziano of the Harvard Medical School reported the results at the American Heart Association's 63rd Scientific Sessions during November 1990 in Dallas. The ongoing clinical trial involving 22,000 male physicians compared the heart disease and stroke incidence of physicians who for six years took either a placebo (inert pill) or beta-carotene without knowing which they were taking.

Dr. William A. Pryor of Louisiana State University was quoted by *Science News* (11/17/90) as stating that this prospective well-controlled study is "the first direct evidence that antioxidant nutrients can counteract atherosclerosis in humans. The Harvard study offers the kind of gold-standard proof that physicians have been waiting for."

Chromium

GTF is a fairly newly discovered nutrient that has been shown by university studies to improve HDL levels by 18%, while decreasing LDL by 18% improving the HDL/LDL ratio by 44%, and lowering the total blood cholesterol by 25%. GTF is thought to be produced in the body from the trace mineral chromium and amino acids, but uncertainty exists about its molecular structure.

Some people do not form as much GTF as they need for optimum health due to diseases such as diabetes, genetic shortcomings, stress, or undernourishment. Such individuals respond well to GTF supplements. Others having efficient GTF production manufacture adequate amounts of GTF once their intake of chromium is optimized. These individuals can improve their HDL/LDL ratios with supplements of either GTF or chromium. Brewer's yeast is a good food source of both GTF and chromium.

At the Federation of American Societies for Experimental Biology meeting in New Orleans on March 21, 1989, Dr. Gary Evans of Bemidji State University (Minnesota) presented the evidence that chromium picolinate reduced total blood cholesterol levels, lowered harmful LDL and apolipoprotein B levels, and increased the "good" HDL and apolipoprotein A levels.

The double-blind crossover study was done jointly with Dr. Raymond I. Press of the Mercy Hospital in San Diego, California and was published in the *Western Journal of Medicine*.[16] The study involved thirty-two subjects and found that 200 micrograms of chromium as 1.6 milligrams of chromium picolinate reduced the "cholesterol number" of persons with moderately elevated cholesterol levels by an average of twenty points (from 276 to 256).

When the subjects taking chromium picolinate switched to the placebo their cholesterol levels gradually returned to their previous values.

The volunteers also had improvements in the more important parameters of the cholesterol–heart disease link. Their "bad" LDL cholesterol dropped by an average of twenty-two points (from 200 to 178) and the "good" HDL cholesterol increased by three points (from 52 to 55). There was no significant effect on triglyceride levels.

The improvement in blood chemistry seems to be brought about by an improvement in the production of the proteins that form the lipoproteins. As discussed earlier, HDL is made largely from apolipoprotein A, while LDL is made largely from apolipoprotein B.

The study found that chromium picolinate enabled the body to produce more HDL-forming apolipoprotein A. Subjects taking the chromium picolinate increased apolipoprotein A levels by 16 milligrams per deciliter (from 147 to 163) while decreasing their apolipoprotein B levels by 25 milligrams per deciliter (from 155 to 130).

The resultant change in the all-important HDL/LDL ratio was from 52/200 to 55/178. This is a 20% improvement of 0.26 to 0.31. This 20% improvement in HDL/LDL ratio is extremely important and may be overlooked by those merely looking at the 7% reduction (19/276 = 0.072) in total cholesterol, which is a fairly meaningless indicator of true risk. The most accurate indicators assessed by blood chemistry are Lp(a) and apolipoprotein B levels, and TC/HDL and HDL/LDL ratios.

Chromium is consumed by sugar metabolism, and more than 90% of Americans do not get the RDA for chromium. Earlier studies had linked low chromium levels with diseased arteries and heart disease.

The fact that GTF often leads to increased HDL levels and thus less risk of heart disease has been reported in the *Journal of the American Medical Association,* the *American Journal of Clinical Nutrition,* and the *Journal of the American College of Nutrition.*

Early studies had shown that persons dying of heart disease have virtually no chromium or silicon in their aortas, whereas those dying from accidents have higher, more normal levels of chromium in their arteries. However, nearly all adult Americans have less chromium in their arteries than inhabitants of those countries where heart disease incidence is low.

Dr. Abraham Abraham of the department of medicine at Shaare Zedak Hospital in Jerusalem has shown that increased amounts of dietary chromium reversed the plaque (so-called "cholesterol deposits") in monkeys. His research group concluded,

> "These experiments have shown that atherosclerosis, even when established, can be reversed by treatment with chromium. After a relatively short treatment period of thirty weeks with chromium there was substantial regression of atherosclerotic lesions, both macroscopically (the aortas weighed less and were freer of plaque) and in terms of cholesterol content, as compared to the group that did not receive chromium. The difference between the extent of aortic involvement in the chromium-treated and non-treated groups was significant by all the methods we used."

An important study was conducted at the Division of Cardiology in Bordeaux-Gradignan, France. Patients having the symptoms of cardiovascular disease were examined by coronary cineangiography. The patients were divided into three groups: those with coronary artery disease (CAD), those with heart disease but no CAD, and those with neither CAD nor heart disease. The CAD and heart disease groups showed lower blood levels of chromium than the disease-free group. Patients whose arteries were relatively free of plaque were found to have three to eight times as much chromium in their blood as those whose arteries were severely blocked.

The researchers concluded that an upper limit for blood levels of chromium could exist beyond which the likelihood of developing CAD or heart disease is improbable.

Also, studies have linked high insulin levels with heart disease. Chromium, and especially GTF, potentiate insulin in such a manner as to normalize blood sugar levels while keeping blood levels of insulin at a minimum.

We can no longer ignore the extensive evidence that is in the literature that demonstrates that chromium is protective against heart disease.

Copper

A copper-deficient diet raises blood cholesterol level, deranges the heart's electrical patterns, and impairs glucose tolerance.

According to Dr. Leslie M. Klevay of the U. S. Department of Agriculture, almost everybody needs more copper. Dr. Klevay has been working on the copper-fat connection at the Human Nutrition Research Center in Grand Forks, North Dakota. He's found that studies *blaming dietary fat* for clogging the hearts of laboratory mice *should actually have blamed a low-copper diet*.

He's noted that for efficient functioning of two enzymes that lower cholesterol, copper is essential. Earlier studies also showed copper essential for glucose tolerance. In other studies Dr. Klevay found that copper-deficient diets produce abnormal electrocardiograms.

Nearly fifty similarities between copper-deficient animals and persons with heart disease have been observed.[17]

Dr. Sheldon Reiser and colleagues fed copper-deficient

diets to twenty-four volunteer men. After eleven weeks their LDL-cholesterol and total cholesterol had increased, while their HDL-cholesterol had decreased.[18]

Niacin

One of the first cholesterol-lowering nutrients tested under sponsorship of the National Heart, Lung and Blood Institute was niacin. It was part of the Coronary Drug Project headed by Dr. Stamler of Northwestern University Medical School. The study found niacin at 3,000 milligrams per day to be very effective, but a side effect experienced by most people at the start of megadosing with niacin was considered a drawback. Now 3,000 milligrams per day is a huge megadose that shouldn't be taken unless the patient is monitored for side effects by a physician! Before we discuss the potent cholesterol-lowering effect of niacin, let's talk a little about these side effects.

One harmless but annoying side effect is a brief, warm, flushing sensation—and sometimes an itch—as niacin causes histamine stored in skin to be released. This niacin flush lasts only momentarily and usually disappears in a few days or weeks of high niacin intake as excess histamine is no longer stored in the skin. However, if someone doesn't know about the niacin flush and takes large doses of niacin, it can scare the devil out of them.

A serious side effect can arise in some persons taking huge amounts of niacin. Niacin lowers cholesterol by interfering with a liver enzyme that helps make cholesterol. Too much interference with the level of this enzyme can damage the liver of some persons. Liver-function tests should be performed by a physician to monitor liver status. This effect has only been reported in a time-release niacin supplement so far, but theoretically, it could occur in standard supplements at high dosage.

Niacin is also called nicotinic acid and vitamin B-3. Another compound with vitamin B-3 activity is niacinamide. Niacinamide can be used in the body to form the same enzymes that niacin can, but niacinamide does not effectively lower blood cholesterol levels, nor does it produce the niacin flush. That is why it is popular. Niacinamide is also called nicotinamide. If you are trying to lower your cholesterol, do not use a product labeled as vitamin B-3 unless it also states that the form of vitamin B-3 is niacin or nicotinic acid.

In a study at Harvard University Medical School, cholesterol was lowered 18% in over one hundred heart patients taking a gram (1,000 mg) of niacin daily. Niacin also improved HDL. A dosage of 1,500 milligrams (1.5 grams) daily can result in a lowering of LDL by 30%. Dosages up to 7,500 milligrams daily have been used to lower blood cholesterol levels an average of 45%. This is too drastic for nonsupervised use and should only be done under the guidance of a physician.

In a follow-up study reported in the *Journal of the American College of Cardiology* of the 8,000 men originally studied in the Coronary Drug Project, there was a huge surprise. The follow-up study found *11% fewer deaths among those who took the niacin!* The original Coronary Drug Project had shown that niacin resulted in about 27 fewer nonfatal heart attacks but had not shown the reduction in deaths. It took several years for the lifesaving results to show up in all of the statistics.

Physicians at the Scientific Institute of Internal Medicine in Genoa, Italy found in 1984 that vitamins A and E were synergistic with niacin in lowering LDL cholesterol and improving HDL.

Lecithin

HDL is manufactured partly from the body's natural emulsifier, lecithin. Nutrients such as polyunsaturated fatty acids, the B-complex vitamins, and the minerals magnesium and phosphorus are used by our bodies in the manufacture of lecithin, a phospholipid. If we are deficient in any of these nutrients, we will not make the right amount of HDL.

Eggs contain cholesterol, but they also contain lecithin. In fact, when you eat eggs your HDL/LDL ratio improves because of the egg lecithin. The "prudent" approach avoids eggs because of cholesterolphobia. The danger in avoiding eggs is that it becomes easier to unbalance the diet. Eggs are very nutritious and, relatively speaking, are not a high-fat food. The high-nutrient-density egg, in moderate amounts, is beneficial to more than 95% of the population. The only ones who should exclude eggs from their diets are those having the genetic imperfection that results in the disease hyper-lipoproteinemia.

Lecithin is also available in supplement form. However, this form of lecithin is usually soybean lecithin, which is slightly different, and slightly less effective, than egg lecithin and the lecithin that can be manufactured in your own body.

However, the benefits of soya lecithin on blood cholesterol levels was studied by researchers at the Technion-Israel Institute of Technology in Haifa, Israel.[19] They found that 12 grams of soya lecithin daily after three months lowered blood cholesterol by 15% and reduced triglycerides by 23%. HDL was increased by 16%.

Fish Oil

A special polyunsaturated fat called eicosapentaenoic acid (EPA), which is found in the oil of cold saltwater fish such as mackerel, herring, and cod, has been found to improve the HDL/LDL ratio significantly and to lower total cholesterol level.

There may be a synergistic effect between calcium and fish oil, according to Dr. David McCarron of the Oregon Health Science University at Portland.

A 1983 Welsh study of over one hundred men placed on a diet that averaged about a half of a gram of EPA per day had an average decrease in blood triglyceride levels. Some physicians believe that high blood triglyceride levels may be a risk factor in heart disease, but there is not a clear consensus. The researcher concluded that the inclusion of moderate amounts of fatty fish in the diet on a long-term basis reduces blood triglyceride levels and may be beneficial in the prevention of heart disease.

Dr. William E. Connor and his colleagues at the Oregon Health Sciences University in Portland have been at the forefront of research on the beneficial effects of fish oil on the heart and arteries. This group has been an influential factor in American research and opinion on the subject since the early 1980s. In 1983 and 1984 they published articles examining another research aspect of the protective effect of fish oils.

Dr. Connor's group examined the effect of fish oil on high-carbohydrate diets. High-carbohydrate diets increase the blood levels of very low density lipoprotein (VLDL) and triglycerides. VLDL are carriers that transport mostly triglycerides and some cholesterol in the blood. VLDL are smaller than the more familiar LDL and HDL. The role of VLDL is not as well understood, but some researchers feel that a high level of VLDL is also a risk factor in heart disease.

The studies compared the effects of fish oils and plant oils on the blood levels of VLDL and triglycerides in healthy persons eating a high-carbohydrate diet. The healthy volunteers were placed on a diet that was 45% carbohydrate and 45% fat for a period of time to establish "normal" baseline measurements. Next they were placed on a 75% carbohydrate diet, having 15% of the diet consisting of peanut oil and cocoa butter. I hope the diet was more palatable than it sounds! After a period of time they were given a diet in which the plant fats were replaced with fish oils, while the remainder of the diet was the same. From the sound of the diet we can conclude that these volunteers made sacrifices for the betterment of science.

When the volunteers consumed the high-carbohydrate diet without the fish oils their blood levels of triglycerides rose an average of 85% while their VLDL more than doubled. When they were switched to the high-carbohydrate diet with fish oils their blood level of triglycerides dropped from the elevated level to a level that was even lower than the baseline level of the moderate-carbohydrate diet. Their average VLDL level dropped 78%, and their cholesterol level dropped 65%, to below baseline level. These effects were seen within three days of adding fish oil to the diet.

The researchers concluded that high triglyceride levels induced by a high-carbohydrate diet can be prevented and reversed by fish oils. They postulated that the mechanism involved was either a reduction in the production of the triglyceride carrier VLDL or improved removal of VLDL from the blood.

In 1985 members of this research group reported that fish oils produced dramatic drops in blood triglyceride levels in patients having highly elevated levels of triglycerides. Fish oils did much better than corn oil or safflower oil.

A study from the University of Karlovy in Praha, Czecho-slovakia also showed that fish oils reduced high triglycerides. Men with elevated blood levels of triglycerides who were given about 18 ounces of fish daily for three months had reductions in triglyceride levels and improvements in HDL levels.

In 1986 Dr. Paul Nestel of the Baker Medical Research Institute in Melbourne, Australia showed that adding fish oil to a high-cholesterol diet prevented an increase in blood cholesterol levels and possibly reduced the risk of heart disease. He fed volunteers three different diets over a seven-week period: a normal diet, a fish-oil diet, and a fish-oil-and-egg-yolk diet.

The normal diet had a polyunsaturated-fat-to-saturated-fat ratio of 0.47 and a daily cholesterol level of 710 milligrams. The fish-oil diet (40 grams of MaxEPA per day) had a PUFA-to-saturated-fat ratio of 1.62 and a daily cholesterol level of 190 milligrams. The fish-oil-and-egg-yolk diet had a PUFA-to-saturated-fat ratio of 1.62 and a daily cholesterol level of 940 milligrams.

When the volunteers were switched from the normal diet to the fish-oil diet their blood cholesterol, VLDL, LDL, HDL, and triglyceride levels declined. When they were then switched to the fish-oil-and-egg-yolk (high cholesterol) diet, the expected elevation in those blood components did not occur; however, cholesterol levels did rise slightly. It was concluded that fish oils are effective in lowering lipoprotein cholesterol levels even when the dietary intake of cholesterol is high.

A research team at the University of Leiden's Institute of Social Medicine in the Netherlands led by Dr. Daan Kromhout produced the first long-term study of the effects of fish oils on heart-disease deaths. The results made a lot of researchers and practicing physicians sit up and take notice.

As the researchers put it, "We were aware of the low death rate from coronary heart disease among the Greenland Eskimos. We therefore decided to investigate the relation between fish consumption and coronary heart disease in a group of men in the town of Zutphen, the Netherlands. Information about the fish consumption of 852 middle-aged men without clinical signs or any other indication of coronary heart disease was collected in 1960 by a careful dietary history obtained from the participants and their wives.

"During twenty years of follow-up, seventy-eight men died from coronary heart disease. An inverse dose-response relation was observed between the consumption in 1960 and the death from coronary heart disease during twenty years of follow-up. This relation persisted after factoring for other variables. Mortality from coronary heart disease was 58% lower among those who consumed at least 30 grams (slightly more than an ounce) of fish per day than among those who did not eat fish.

"We conclude that the consumption of as little as one or two fish dishes per week may be of preventive value in relation to coronary heart disease."

The relationship existed throughout the time period. Twenty-seven men died from coronary heart disease between 1960 and 1970, fifty-one between 1971 and 1980. The more fish the men ate, the less death due to heart disease, and the lower the total death rate, as other diseases were not affected.

For those who worry too much about dietary cholesterol, it should be noted that the men eating the most fish also ate the most cholesterol and animal protein, yet they had fewer heart-disease deaths. Please keep in mind the studies showing that fish and fish oils both tend to lower blood cholesterol levels, regardless of the dietary cholesterol content.

On September 26, 1985 the *New England Journal of Medicine* published some of the letters it had received commenting on the three articles and the editorial in the May 9 issue. Among the responses was data from the group that conducted the Western Electric study on heart disease that began in 1957. When Drs. Jeremiah Stamler, Richard Shekelle, Paul Oglesby, et al. examined their data in terms of fish consumption versus heart-disease death rate, they confirmed the Kromhout, et al. observations. The Western Electric data showed that the twenty-five-year risk of death from coronary heart disease was only 65% for those men consuming more than thirty-five grams of fish per day as an average compared to those who did not eat fish.

Wheat Germ Oil

It may turn out that wheat germ oil may be at least as beneficial as fish oil, and possibly better. It's too early to tell, as there has been only one study at this writing. In a comparison of four fats in high-fat diets at the University of Chicago, Dr. Robert Wissler and his colleagues found that wheat germ oil and fish oil permitted only one-third the rise in total blood cholesterol observed in high-fat diets where the fat was coconut oil or crude menhaden fish oil. However, wheat germ oil improved HDL levels the most and improved clotting time the best.

Gamma-linolenic acid

Gamma-linolenic acid (GLA) is an omega-one type of dietary polyunsaturated fatty acid. It is used in the body to make the "good" prostaglandins of the PG-1 family. Like the PG-3 family of prostaglandins formed from the omega-three polyunsaturated fatty acid EPA, the PG-1 prostaglandins control many body reactions that are beneficial.

Evening primrose oil, borage oil, and black currants are rich sources of GLA. Other seeds also contain smaller levels of GLA.

Japanese researchers gave volunteers with high LDL-cholesterol levels 3.6 grams of evening primrose oil for eight weeks. They found no adverse effects and confirmed that evening primrose oil is effective in lowering LDL in patients with high levels.[20]

An earlier Japanese study had found that evening primrose oil had a greater cholesterol-lowering effect than all other unsaturated oils tested, including safflower oil and olive oil.[21]

Vitamin E

Dr. William Hermann of the Methodist Hospital in Houston found that vitamin E increased HDL levels by 15% and lowered LDL levels by 10% in only six weeks. Although one study failed to confirm this, two other independent studies have done so. The one study that failed to confirm this study was designed to detect only HDL increases above 50% because an earlier but very small study had reported a 400% improvement.

Dr. Stuart Hartz of Tufts University has determined that HDL is higher among vitamin E–supplement users in an epidemiological survey.

After further study, Dr. Hermann concluded that the effects of vitamin E on people with normal HDLs are variable. However, when HDL is less than 15% of the total cholesterol, vitamin E is very effective in improving HDL. Also, above thirty-five years of age, vitamin E has less of an effect.[22]

A 1987 study found that 500 IU of vitamin E daily for three months produced a significantly improved HDL cholesterol level, Apo A level, and Apo A/Apo B ratio.[23]

Drs. Thomas Muckle and Darius Nazir were intrigued with the fact that fifteen published studies showed that vitamin E improved HDL and nine studies found no effect, so they did their own study in 1989.[24]

Eight healthy adults were given 800 IU of vitamin E daily for sixty-four days. HDL levels rose in six of the volunteers beginning ten to fourteen days after starting the vitamin E supplements. The results were significant and lasting in three of the volunteers.

Dr. W. L. Stone and colleagues have shown that animals on vitamin E- and selenium-deficient diets have elevated LDL levels that can be corrected by supplementation.[25]

Low levels of vitamins C and E correlate with increased incidence of heart disease.[26]

Vitamin C

As long ago as 1965, Dr. Emil Ginter, director of the Research Institute of Human Nutrition in Bratislava, Czechoslovakia established that low blood levels of vitamin C elevated blood cholesterol levels and increased the amount of cholesterol in artery plaque.

Seasonal variations in a person's blood cholesterol level can often be traced to seasonal variation in dietary vitamin C.

Vitamin C can also improve the HDL cholesterol level and TC/HDL ratio, according to a study at Tufts University's Human Nutrition Research Center on Aging. Dr. Stuart Hartz and colleagues found that HDL began improving with a vitamin C level above 120 milligrams daily. Further improvement was noted at higher vitamin C intakes. At a gram (1,000 mg.) daily there was an 8% increase in HDL compared to those consuming less than 120 milligrams daily.

Another study in Boston found that vitamin C increased HDL in women and nonsmoking men. Vitamin C improved apolipoprotein A-1 in all persons.[27]

The British medical journal *Lancet* has commented that two studies have shown that in people with high blood cholesterol given 300 milligrams, 450 milligrams, or one gram of vitamin C per day there were decreases in LDL and total blood cholesterol.

A 1985 study by Drs. L. Chen and R. Thayer of the University of Kentucky also confirms this effect.[28]

Keep in mind that smokers have less vitamin C in their blood than nonsmokers at any given level of vitamin C intake.

In 1986 Dr. T. Bazzarre of the University of North Carolina found that 1,000 milligrams (one gram) of vitamin C daily decreased blood cholesterol in both smokers and nonsmokers.[29] HDL levels were increased more in the nonsmokers. Vitamin C blood levels in the smokers were lower even though they received the same dose of supplement.

Importantly, Dr. Bazzarre found that the higher the blood cholesterol level, the lower the total blood cholesterol level, and vice versa. He also found that vitamin C was more effective in those with blood cholesterol levels above 250 than in those with lower cholesterol.

A combination of vitamins C and E protected arteries against cholesterol deposits when high amounts of cholesterol were fed to monkeys.[30]

Earlier in this chapter (see p. 168) we noted that vitamin C lowers the "bad" lipoprotein Lp(a).

Fiber

Some dietary fibers have improved HDL/LDL ratios. Fibers also lower the total cholesterol level of the blood because they increase the production of bile, which is made from cholesterol. This says a lot for a high-fiber diet, but if you choose to eat a low-fiber diet, keep in mind that you can obtain much of the benefit by taking mixed-fiber or bran supplements.

There are two main physical categories of fiber—soluble and insoluble—and five chemical classes of fibers—cellulose, hemicelluloses, gums, pectin, and lignin—and you should have ample amounts of each in your diet.

Soluble fibers can help lower high blood cholesterol levels, and insoluble fibers can decrease transit time.

Cellulose increases bulk, softens stools, relieves constipation, counteracts bowel carcinogens, modulates blood sugar level, and helps control appetite. Cellulose has no known effect on blood cholesterol level. Excellent sources are fruits, vegetables, bran, seeds, nuts, and beans.

Hemicelluloses increase bulk, relieve constipation, counteract bowel carcinogens, and help control appetite. Their effects are very similar to those of cellulose, and they are found in the same foods.

Gums lower blood cholesterol and modulate blood sugar levels. Good food sources of gums are oats, barley, and dried beans. Pectins lower blood cholesterol, counter bowel bile acids, and offer some protection against bowel cancer and gallstones. Gums and pectins are water soluble and thus do not hold water. Therefore they have no effect on stool bulk and constipation. Good food sources for pectins are carrots, apples, prunes, citrus fruits, and, contrary to popular opinion, bran.

Lignins increase removal of cholesterol and bile acids from the bowel, thereby protecting against bowel cancer and gallstones. Good sources are prunes, cereals, bran, fruits, and vegetables.

Good fibers for lowering cholesterol include oat bran, psyllium seeds, beans, guar gum, carrot pectin, rice bran, and citrus fruits. If you can't switch to a diet rich in fiber, you may wish to add fiber supplements to your present diet.

Table 17.6 is a guide to indicate which foods have which types of fiber, and Table 17.7 indicates the effect some fibers have on blood cholesterol levels.

TABLE 17.6
Fibers and Their Effects

Good Cancer Protection (Insoluble Fiber)	(Both)	Good Heart Protection (Soluble Fiber)
Wheat bran	Kidney beans	Apples
Wheat products	Navy beans	Bananas
Brown rice	Green beans	Citrus fruits
Cooked lentils	Green peas	Carrots
	Pinto beans	Barley
		Oats
		Rice bran

TABLE 17.7
Effect of Fiber on Cholesterol

Fiber	Quantity g/day	% decrease in blood cholesterol
Cellulose	16	0
Wheat bran	17	0
Whole oats	15	11
Oat bran	27	17
Pectin	25	13
Guar gum	24	16
Beans	30	19
Psyllium seed	10	15

Oat Bran

Studies showing that oats lower blood cholesterol go back to Dr. A. P. DeGroot in 1963, but oat bran didn't reach its great popularity until 1988.[31-40] A study in 1990 involving twenty persons having normal blood cholesterol levels indicated that the positive effect was not due to the soluble fiber but instead was because the oats replaced fats in the diet.[41] The criticism is that this study only involved twenty people, which is enough for statistical significance only if the people were all identical and everything went as planned (which it never seems to do). Another criticism is that the study was with normal-cholesterol persons, not those with high cholesterol. More testing is needed to clarify the issue.

Dr. James Anderson of the University of Kentucky has found that the soluble fiber in oat bran can lower blood cholesterol levels as much as ten percent. Dr. Anderson believes that oats (whole oats contain bran too) can lower blood cholesterol levels more than a low-fat diet can.[42]

There are about 6.3 grams of soluble fiber in every 100 grams of oat bran, and about 5 grams of soluble fiber in every 100 grams of oatmeal. An effective amount of oat bran is about 50 to 100 grams daily, which will provide about three to six grams of soluble fiber (an ounce is about 28 grams).

Adding oat bran to your diet is fairly simple. Start by adding one-third cup daily for a week, then two thirds of a cup daily for another week, and finally go for the long run with a cup of oat bran cereal every two or three days. Variety is the spice of life, so don't make oat bran cereal a daily event. You need other foods as well for balanced nutrition and to keep the oat bran cereal fresh-tasting for the long haul.

Try eating pinto or navy beans on the days you don't eat oat bran cereal. Remember that other forms of fiber such as wheat bran are needed for cancer protection.

Psyllium Fiber

Dr. Anderson also found that three tablespoons of psyllium seed husks reduced total blood cholesterol levels by an average of 15% in thirteen men studied and, importantly, reduced LDL cholesterol by an average of 20%.[43]

Psyllium seed husks have been commonly used as a laxative for more than fifty years. They are a rich source of soluble fiber but also contain ample insoluble fiber. Psyllium fiber is water-holding, so it softens stools. It moderates emptying of the stomach and thus suppresses the appetite. Psyllium fiber also adds bulk to increase bacterial fermentation and enhances bile acid secretion.

Ounce for ounce, psyllium fiber contains five times more soluble fiber than oat bran or wheat bran. Psyllium fiber is 80% soluble, compared to less than 15% solubility of oat bran and wheat bran on an equal-weight basis.

Gamma-oryzanol

Rice bran is also getting a lot of attention for lowering cholesterol, but the real active ingredient is believed to be gamma-oryzanol. The scientific literature shows that gamma-oryzanol inhibits cholesterol absorption, inhibits cholesterol deposition in arteries, and increases HDL production. Gamma-oryzanol is actually a mixture of ferulic acid derivatives from rice, and is an antioxidant. Its safety has been demonstrated by over twenty-five years of use in Japan.

In a study led by Dr. G. Yoshino, sixty-seven patients having high cholesterol were given 300 milligrams of gamma-oryzanol daily. After two months the average blood cholesterol decrease was 89%, and after three months the average blood cholesterol decrease was 12%.

Beta-sitosterol

For those individuals who do absorb dietary cholesterol efficiently with a resultant increase in blood cholesterol, beta sitosterol will be of interest. Vegetarian diets are not only extremely low in cholesterol, they are rich in a compound that is similar in structure to cholesterol, but different in function. This compound is beta-sitosterol. The chemical similarity allows the compound to be absorbed and carried by the same system that transports cholesterol. The result is that beta-sitosterol blocks the absorption of cholesterol.

Beta-sitosterol is a member of a class of steroid compounds called phytosterols. Other members found in the diet in smaller amounts include campesterol and stigmosterols. The latter compounds are steroids, too, but not as similar to cholesterol, and thus they do not block cholesterol absorption as well as beta-sitosterol. Beta-sitosterol is most effective when taken just prior to a meal so that it can block the cholesterol in the meal from being absorbed.

Research performed as long ago as 1953 has shown that beta-sitosterol lowers blood cholesterol levels.[44] Later, Canadian researchers showed that 300 milligrams of beta-sitosterol daily significantly lowered blood cholesterol.[45] In 1982 researchers showed that beta-sitosterol taken as a supplement controls blood cholesterol levels in many persons without a change in diet.[46] The role of beta-sitosterol in controlling blood cholesterol level was discussed in *Nutrition Reviews* in 1987.[47]

Charcoal

Another cholesterol blocker is powdered "activated" charcoal. A tablespoon of powdered activated charcoal taken after every meal can reduce blood cholesterol by 20% to 25% in those persons responsive to cholesterol absorption. A Finnish study showed that a quarter ounce of activated charcoal after each meal for a month *lowered LDL cholesterol by 41%!*

Dr. Eli A. Friedman of the SUNY Health Science Center in Brooklyn found that 35 grams (an ounce is 28 grams) of charcoal daily *lowered total cholesterol by 43% and triglycerides by 76%!*

The activated charcoal's many pores act as a filter to remove many undesired compounds. It can also remove some important nutrients, so be sure to supplement your diet if you use activated charcoal regularly.

Garlic

Garlic reduces total blood cholesterol and triglyceride levels by 10% to 30% and can raise blood HDL-cholesterol levels by as much as 30%.[48]

Dimethylglycine

The amino acid dimethylglycine (DMG) is a nonfuel nutrient and metabolite. DMG's role in cancer protection was discussed in Chapter 12. In a group of fourteen patients with high cholesterol there was an average drop of forty-one points (12%) over nine months with DMG. Their HDL levels were also improved. Three of the patients were nonresponsive and had no change in their total blood cholesterol levels or HDL levels. If these three persons were omitted from the averages, the average drop would have been fifty-two points (16%).

In clinical evaluations by Dr. Mitchell Pries of over 400 geriatric cardiovascular patients there was major improvement in the following areas with DMG:

1. increase in feeling of well-being, vitality, and mobility
2. improvement in circulatory insufficiency
3. decrease in high blood cholesterol
4. reduction in angina pain
5. fewer irregular heartbeats
6. decrease of high blood pressure
7. improvement in heart response to stress tests

L-Carnitine

L-Carnitine is an amino acid-like compound that does not enter into protein structures. Its purpose is to help muscle cells, especially heart cells, use fats for energy. L-carnitine helps carry fats into the mitochondria, the power plants of cells, and stimulates the oxidation of the fats to produce energy.

As people age they tend to produce less L-carnitine. Good diets may keep us adequately nourished in L-carnitine, but poor diets may produce a deficiency severe enough to allow fats to build up in the blood. This will tend to raise triglycerides and LDL levels.

Supplementation with L-carnitine can normalize these factors when an L-carnitine deficiency was the cause of their elevation.[49]

Taurine

The amino acid taurine is widely researched in Japan and is a popular food supplement because it lowers cholesterol, normalizes blood pressure, and strengthens the heart.

It is not surprising that taurine lowers blood cholesterol, because it plays an important role in bile formation. Cholesterol and taurine combine with other compounds to form bile. If there is not enough taurine, then less cholesterol will be used to form bile. With extra taurine, bile production can proceed to capacity, and more cholesterol will be consumed in the process. Dr. Yukio Yamori of the Shimane Medical University in Izumo, Japan confirms that taurine supplements can lower blood cholesterol after four weeks of use.[50]

Mucopolysaccharides

Mucopolysaccharides (MPS) are complex carbohydrates that lower LDL while increasing HDL.[51] MPS also improve the integrity of arteries and capillaries. MPS are recommended by Dr. Lester Morrison for both prevention and treatment of heart disease. MPS are discussed in more detail in Chapter 20 on treating heart disease.

Alcohol Does *Not* Help

Previously, several surveys had indicated that moderate drinking of alcohol resulted in fewer heart-disease deaths than heavy drinking or abstinence. Further, it was shown that one or two alcoholic beverages a day elevated HDL and thus improved the HDL/LDL ratio. However, this is not quite accurate. The HDL fraction that is improved—the HDL-2—does not protect against heart disease. This fraction is an unimportant component of the HDL family. Recent studies confirm that alcohol in any amount harms the heart by enlarging the left ventricle. More than two drinks a day causes considerable damage to the heart.

That's the bad news. The good news is that you shouldn't put too much stock in one study, especially when there are studies that indicate otherwise.

I feel that the body can handle anything in moderation. "The poison is not the compound, but the dose" is an old Latin proverb that pharmacy students are taught. I also believe that a quiet meal with a glass of wine helps friends relax, and that reduces stress and improves body chemistry. And I am a total teetotaler.

However, the new information should be considered. The 1989 study examined the experiences of men in the ongoing Framingham study. The study was presented to the American Heart Association meeting in New Orleans on November 14, 1989. It suggests that even a drink or two puts middle-age men at risk for heart failure and death.

The left ventricle is the heart's main pumping chamber. Left ventricle enlargement is associated with dangerous irregular heart rhythms. The more the ventricle size increases, the greater the risk of heart failure and death. The more alcohol consumed, the more ventricular enlargement. The effect is very dose-dependent and holds true at all dose levels.

Dr. Teri Manolio of the National Heart, Lung and Blood Institute noted, "Anyone past the page of fifty or so, and certainly anyone who already has an enlarged heart, would be better off not drinking at all."

The risk of death increases with the number of drinks per day, age, obesity, and blood pressure. So if you already have risk factors, alcohol increases the risk. Other studies have shown that alcohol is toxic to heart cells and brain cells and that it increases blood pressure.

Or to put it more scientifically, the benefit-to-risk ratio decreases. Although several studies still show apparent benefit in moderate drinking, it may be an effect of relaxation rather than one of HDL improvement. It seems that the HDL improvement is in HDL-2, a fraction of HDL that seems to be of no benefit.

Supplements

If you are worried about your diet and heart disease, go to your physician or clinic and ask to have your TC/HDL ratio determined. If it is okay, then don't worry about this aspect of heart disease and diet (the normal values will be indicated with your test results). If your LDL is too high or your TC/HDL ratio is poor, then discuss the merits of changing to either the "prudent" or "alternative" strategy with your doctor. If, after consultation with your health advisors, you decide that your best bet is the alternative strategy, then consider the following supplements to optimize your TC/HDL ratio.

You won't have to take all of these supplements. It's just that different people have different nutritional deficiencies. Also, there is the matter of biochemical individuality. Start with what seems reasonable to you based on what you are missing most in your diet and which you can tolerate well. Make adjustments as you progress based on your blood analysis.

As an example, you may wish to add soluble fibers to your diet and take chromium picolinate, antioxidant nutrients, copper, and taurine as supplements. That should do the job for most people.

TABLE 17.8
Lowering Your Cholesterol

Nutrient	Daily Amount
Glucose tolerance factor (GTF) (or 100 micrograms of chromium) *or*	25–50 mcg
Chromium picolinate	1–2 mg
Copper	1–2 mg
Beta-carotene	15,000–30,000 USP
Fish oil (EPA)	4–8 g
Wheat germ oil	500 mg–1 g
Vitamin C	500–5,000 mg
Vitamin E	400–800 IU
Lecithin	as labeled
Fiber	as labeled
Niacin	250 mg (1,000–3,000 mg under doctor's monitoring)
Dimethylglycine	100–200 mg
Gamma-oryzanol	300 mg
Beta-sitosterol	300 mg
"Activated" charcoal	tablespoon after meals
Garlic	1–2 capsules
Gamma-linolenic acid (GLA)	1–3 grams
L-carnitine	500–1,000 mg
Taurine	1,000–3,000 mg
Mucopolysaccharides (MPS)	as labeled

If you wish to lower your cholesterol more, you can consider adding more fiber as a supplement and also include niacin. That should take care of just about everybody. On the other hand, some people may experience uncomfortable bloating and cramps from the fiber and wish to cut back on fiber and substitute charcoal or fish oil.

You should try different combinations that best suit your preferences for diet and supplements while regularly monitoring your TC/HDL ratio. Work with your physician and all health care professionals as partners. They are your advisors, but the ultimate responsibility for your health rests with you.

If you are on drugs to "thin your blood" or increase your clotting time, do not start supplementation without your physician's knowledge or you may decrease the clotting time too much. Check back with your doctor at two-month intervals, or as otherwise directed, to monitor your progress in optimizing your TC/HDL ratio.

18

Preventing Heart Attacks

The foregoing chapter was concerned with preventing arterial disease (cholesterol deposits or fatty plaques). What is the alternative strategy for one who already has narrowed arteries? After all, nearly everyone is walking around with at least a fair degree of narrowing.

This chapter contains information on how to keep your blood flowing freely through your arteries even when they are narrowed by cholesterol deposits. Following chapters will discuss how to keep your heart strong, special protection if you smoke, and nutritional support if you already have heart disease.

Heart attacks are caused by blood clots forming in the narrowed arteries of the heart (coronary arteries). This is called coronary thrombosis. The blood clots shut off the flow of blood to heart tissue, which then dies because of a lack of oxygen. The dead heart tissue is called "myocardial infarction." The severity of the blood clot is determined by both the area of the infarct and the exact tissue destroyed. If the myocardial infarction was not fatal, then scar tissue replaces the infarct. This scar is a patch that enables the heart to return to normal function if it is small enough and not in an extremely critical area.

Infarcts can also be caused by spasms of the coronary arteries that clamp off the flow of blood. Perhaps as many as 20% of fatal heart attacks are caused by artery spasms—even in normal, plaque-free arteries.

While it is true that narrowed arteries cause physical damage to blood cells called "platelets" that increase the tendency of the blood to clot, there are other causes of undesirable blood clotting in coronary arteries. High-fat diets and nutritional deficiencies can increase this clotting tendency. Conversely, other nutrients can normalize a tendency for the blood to clot. Vitamin E and fish oil (EPA) have been shown to speed the repair of platelet cells that have been damaged by narrowed arteries. Gamma-linolenic acid (GLA), found in evening primrose oil and other sources, also affects prostaglandin balance to help keep the blood slippery.

Blood clotting can also be caused by impairment of fibrinolytic activity, which involves a multistep process beyond the platelet stage.

Vitamin E

In the preceding chapter we examined how vitamin E protects the arteries and showed that low vitamin E levels in the blood are a better predictor of heart disease development than any other parameter. Now let's consider the fact that natural vitamin E has been shown to keep blood slippery by inhibiting a chemical called "platelet phospholipase A-2," according to studies made by Drs. Alvin C. Chan and Carmela Luttinger-Basch of the University of Ottawa. This is a stereochemical property of natural vitamin E (d-alpha-tocopherol or RRR-alpha-tocopherol) that is not shared by the other compounds present in synthetic vitamin E (d,l-alpha-tocopherol or all-rac-alpha-tocopherol).

Another set of studies that shows synthetic vitamin E ineffective and natural vitamin E effective is discussed in Chapter 24 on cystic mastitis. I know there are some who say there is no difference between natural and synthetic vitamin E. The difference has been proven many times with vitamin E. The molecules are different. They are different compounds having many of the same chemical properties, but not all.

It is interesting to note that what makes the blood less likely to clot is altering the ratio of certain prostaglandins. Prostaglandins are hormonelike compounds having great biological influence. They control or influence many body processes, including blood clotting, blood pressure, blood sugar level, menstrual cramps, gastrointestinal secretion, fertility, reproduction, immunity, inflammation, and pain. Other similar compounds called thromboxanes and leukotrienes can be formed from prostaglandins. A prostaglandin called prostacyclin (PGI2) helps prevent blood clotting, while a thromboxane called thromboxane A2 (TXA2) can cause blood to clot. An enzyme called cyclooxygenase helps convert the fatty acid arachidonic acid into prostaglandins, thromboxanes, and leukotrienes normally in a ratio that encourages blood clotting.

Aspirin inhibits the production of prostaglandins and related compounds that favor blood clotting by inhibiting the enzyme cyclooxygenase. If too much aspirin is consumed, there can be a danger that clotting is inhibited so much that internal bleeding can occur.

Aha! You see what's coming. Yes, vitamin E is also involved in prostaglandin formation and can affect blood clotting. The difference is that vitamin E tends to normalize clotting; i.e., vitamin E restores blood clotting to normal, whereas aspirin can lead to serious side effects. My second point is that vitamin E is much safer than aspirin and works better to restore blood to its proper clotting time without overshoot. To drive the safety point home, we all know of aspirin overdose killing (salicylate poisoning), but there is no such thing as a lethal vitamin E overdose. However, aspirin may be beneficial to you.

We'll examine aspirin in more detail in Chapter 20. Right now, let's get back to vitamin E.

Vitamin E modulates the production of prostaglandins at a number of different points, but contrary to some early studies, vitamin E does not inhibit cyclooxygenase. Vitamin E elevates the levels of the anticlotting prostacyclin by blocking the inhibitory effects of lipid peroxides on prostacyclin synthetase. Studies have shown that a vitamin E deficiency results in increased blood platelet (small plate-shaped cells that cause clotting) aggregation (stickier blood) and increased clotting, which can be normalized with vitamin E supplementation.[1]

An additional mechanism has been postulated for high concentrations of vitamin E. Vitamin E can also act as a surfactant (a substance that makes things slippery) that alters the blood platelet membrane. After several studies Drs. Rao Panganamala and David Cornwell conclude that vitamin E can have profound effects in physiological states that are associated with platelet aggregation.

Too few scientists and virtually no physicians are aware of this because they have been repeatedly told that clinical studies proved that vitamin E has no effect on heart disease. No thought is given to the fact that the studies were not designed properly, mainly because of too few patients, too little vitamin E, too short a time, and not knowing what to measure. If a clinical trial were conducted today with the same design used in the aspirin study, it would be clearly demonstrated that vitamin E significantly reduces heart attacks. In fact, I demonstrated this in 1974 with a retrospective clinical study.

My 1974 study involved 17,894 participants who had taken various amounts of vitamin E for varying periods of time. The heart disease rate of these participants was compared to that of the general population having identical ages. In all instances where persons consumed 400 IU or more daily of vitamin E for more than two years, their rate of heart disease was significantly lower than normal (3 per 100, compared to 32 per 100). The amount of heart disease in any age group decreased proportionally with the length of time that vitamin E had been taken. In fact, the length of time was more important than dosage after a minimum of 400 IU daily was taken.

A second finding was that 1,200 IU or more of vitamin E daily for four years or more reduced the incidence of heart disease from 32 per hundred to 10 per hundred persons.

The observation that length of time taking vitamin E is strongly associated with reduced heart disease is strong statistically. The Spearman-Rho statistical association value was 0.96, where 1.00 is perfect association. The correlation is significantly different from zero or chance occurrence at the 0.01 level.

Eighty percent of those with angina pectoris or tachycardia are substantially helped within the first year of use of vitamin E. Figure 18.1 and Tables 18.1 through 18.3 summarize my results.

In more recent clinical trials vitamin E produced a significant reduction of platelet aggregation. In a study of healthy adult volunteers there was a significant reduction in platelet adhesion stimulated by four aggregating surfaces (fibrinogen, fibronectin, collagen I, and collagen V) after two weeks of supplementation with 400 IU of vitamin E daily.[2-4]

In 1986 a Danish study showed that vitamin E inhibits platelet aggregation induced by aggregating agents.[5] The

Figure 18.1

YEARS TAKING VITAMIN E VS HEART DISEASE INCIDENCE

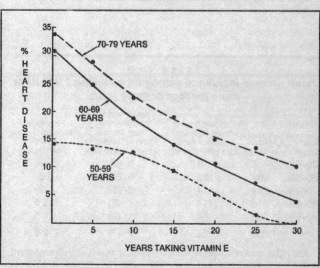

There is a strong correlation between length of time taking vitamin E and freedom from heart disease in all age groups.

TABLE 18.1
Heart disease incidence among those taking 400 IU or more of vitamin E for ten years or more

Age Group	Number in Group	Expected Number with Heart Disease (National Rate from HEW Figures)	Actual Reported Number with Heart Disease (Possible Undetected Cases in Parentheses)	Percentage of Expected Number with Heart Disease
50–59	569	114	0 (3)	0
60–69	871	279	3 (1)	1.1
70–79	806	323	1 (2)	0.3
80–89	245	111	0 (1)	0
90–98	17	9	0 (0)	0
total	2,508	836	4 (7)	0.5

400 IU or more of vitamin E taken for 10 years or more is strongly associated with reduction of the incidence of heart disease prior to 80 years of age to less than 10 percent of the present rate (32 per 100 people expected to have heart disease reduced to 3 per 100 people who actually do have heart disease).

TABLE 18.2
Heart disease incidence among those taking 1,200 IU or more for four or more years

Age Group	Number in Group	Expected Number with Heart Disease (National Rate from HEW Figures)	Actual Reported Number with Heart Disease (Possible Undetected Cases in Parentheses)	Percentage of Expected Number with Heart Disease
90–98	1	0	0 (0)	—
80–89	64	28	0 (0)	0
70–79	284	114	2 (2)	1.8
60–69	356	114	4 (3)	3.5
50–59	333	67	1 (2)	1.5
	1,038	323	7 (7)	2.2

1200 IU or more of vitamin E taken for 4 years or more is strongly associated with reducing the incidence of heart disease prior to 80 years of age from 32 per 100 people to 10 per 100 people.

TABLE 18.3
Correlation between length of time taking vitamin E and freedom from heart disease

Years of Use of Vitamin E Age Group	0	Less than 1	1–3	4–5	6–9	10–19	20–29	30+	Avg.
			Percentage Free from Heart Disease						
50–59	85.7	86.6	86.1	86.2	86.7	89.2	98.3	100	86.8
60–69	68.4	69.6	73.0	74.9	78.7	85.5	89.1	100	76.1
70–79	67.8	64.6	69.1	71.0	70.7	82.1	81.8	88.5	73.6
80–89	65.2	71.8	69.3	67.5	66.9	81.2	85.6	100	73.3
90–98	87.5	100	94.8	77.8	91.7	96.8	—	100	93.4

The association between length of time taking vitamin E and freedom from heart disease is extremely strong statistically. The association (Spearman–Rho) is, in fact, stronger for vitamin E than any other tested variables, which included exercise, diet, and cholesterol intake. The association varies slightly with age, but typically shows a 0.96 association where 1.00 is a perfect association. This correlation is significantly different from chance occurrence at the 0.01 level.

Eighty percent of those with angina pectoris, fibrillation, or tachycardia are substantially helped by tocopherol within the first year of use. Most patients find that they can gradually reduce other medication with increasing time and dosage of vitamin E.

study indicated that vitamin E was especially effective in increasing the production of lipoxygenase products in blood platelets. It also suggested that vitamin E does not have an effect on the arachidonic acid cascade as many believe.

In another study with human volunteers, vitamin E proved to inhibit platelet aggregation induced by ADP, epinephrine, collagen, and arachidonic acid.[6]

A longtime researcher in this field, Dr. Manfred Steiner of Brown University in Rhode Island, and his research group concluded, "Based on our results, we suggest that 400 IU per day may be a near optimal dose of vitamin E to reduce platelet adhesivity. . . . We believe that our studies give convincing evidence of the antiadhesive properties of vitamin E supplementation of the diet. It was especially gratifying that 'reasonable' doses of vitamin E that had no untoward side effects were able to accomplish such reduction."[7]

Vitamin C

Researchers at the Central Institute for Heart and Circulation Research in Berlin found that one gram of vitamin C daily normalized blood platelet adhesion and reduced the interaction of platelets with arterial walls.[8]

When one gram of vitamin C is added to high-fat diets the tendency for the blood platelets to stick together is prevented. In a group of twenty patients with coronary artery disease, treatment with one gram of vitamin C every eight hours for ten days significantly decreased platelet adhesiveness and platelet aggregation.[9]

Garlic

A compound in garlic, cycloalliin, increases fibrinolytic activity by 24% to 130%. Other sulfur-containing compounds in garlic normalize blood platelet adhesion.[10]

Vitamin B-6

An Italian research group has shown that vitamin B-6 affects blood platelet aggregation. When volunteers were given vitamin B-6 supplements their blood platelet adhesion index improved. When the vitamin B-6 supplements were discontinued the volunteers' blood returned to previous values.[11]

Bromelain

An enzyme from pineapples is also a potent inhibitor of platelet aggregation. The mechanism is probably via plasminogen activation.[12] Bromelain has been found to have other helpful roles in preventing and treating heart disease. These roles are reviewed in detail by Dr. Hans Nieper of Germany.[13]

Magnesium

Nutrients such as the mineral magnesium and the amino acid tryptophan have also been shown to prevent the artery spasms that can lead to heart attacks. Magnesium is involved in the artery's relaxation from the pulse-synchronization contractions in response to the heart's electrical signals.

The heart condition called "variant angina" results when the coronary arteries go into spasm. Magnesium supplementation relieves this condition.[14]

Magnesium is also required to keep the heart beating. This role of magnesium will be discussed in the next chapter.

Selenium

Patients suffering death from sudden, first heart attacks were found to be very low in blood selenium levels according to a Dutch study published in the *Journal of the American Medical Association*.[15,16] Their body selenium level as measured by the selenium in their toenails showed that those in the lowest quarter of the levels found in the general population produced a 4.5 times greater incidence of fatal heart attacks. Dr. Frans Kok and colleagues concluded, "The heart attack victims had long-term low selenium levels, indicated by low toenail selenium levels, which probably led to increased risk for a coronary event."

Low blood selenium levels were linked to heart disease by researchers at Finland's University of Kuopio and National Public Health Institute.[17] The study of over a thousand middle-aged men, led by Dr. J. Salonen, found that low blood selenium levels were linked with stickier blood (enhanced platelet aggregability), low HDL, and abnormal exercise electrocardiograms.

A German study showed that persons having heart attacks have low blood selenium blood levels.[18] The low selenium levels were present before the heart attack and were not caused by the heart attack. The University of Mainz researchers, led by Dr. O. Oster, concluded, "The results of this study indicate that low blood selenium levels might be a risk factor for the development of coronary heart disease and might increase the damage to heart tissue from a myocardial infarction."

Mucopolysaccharides (MPS)

Mucopolysaccharides (MPS) are important components in connective tissue and artery tissue. MPS play a major role in the integrity of tissues and their permeability to mineral exchange. MPS also control the electrical charge on the surface of blood platelets. MPS help keep all blood platelets negatively charged so that they repel each other.

Supplements to Prevent Heart Attacks

Thus if you can keep your blood free-flowing in your coronary arteries, you will have no heart attacks. The slipperiness of the blood is measured as the blood platelet adhesion index. When you have your TC/HDL ratio measured, have your blood platelet adhesion index measured as well. If it is in the ideal range, then all is well (normal values will be indicated with the test results). However, you may wish to be sure that you are getting adequate magnesium to prevent artery spasms from occurring. We have no indicator of this probability as yet.

If your blood platelet adhesion index shows that your blood is sticky or has a tendency to clot, then you may wish to discuss with your health professional whether you should take the "prudent" approach and switch to a low-fat diet, or take the "alternative" approach. If you decide that the alternative strategy is your best bet, then consider that EPA, tryptophan, vitamin E, and magnesium are all available as food supplements and are found in most health food stores and drugstores. It is difficult to change to foods rich in these nutrients, as many of the nutrients are newly discovered and are not found in food tables. Remember, you may achieve the best results by combining the prudent and alternative approaches.

The following ranges are frequently used and may be a reasonable starting point for you. After you have been supplementing your diet for six to eight weeks, check back with your physician to monitor your progress toward normalization of your blood platelet adhesion index. If you are already on medication to "thin your blood" or increase your clotting time, then don't start using these supplements without your physician's knowledge. The drugs and the supplements together may make you bleed too easily and not clot properly.

TABLE 18.4
Preventing Heart Attacks

Nutrient	Daily Amount
Vitamin E	400–800 mg
Vitamin C	500–1,000 mg
Vitamin B-6	50–100 mg
Bromelain	500–1,000 mg
Selenium	50–200 mcg
Magnesium	400–600 mg
Eicosapentaenoic acid (EPA)	4–8 g
Gamma-linolenic acid (GLA)	500–1,000 mg
L-tryptophan	500–750 mg
Mucopolysaccharides (MPS)	100–500 mg
Pycnogenol	50–150 mg

Counteracting Adverse Cardiovascular Effects of Smoking

Protecting the lungs is only half the problem for smokers. The heart and arteries must also be protected. Cigarette smoke contains not only carcinogens but also nicotine, carbon monoxide, and other chemicals. Nicotine alters the circulation of blood and increases blood pressure. Carbon monoxide ties up the red blood cells so that they can't deliver enough oxygen. Aldehydes and other chemicals from smoke cause harm to arteries. These chemical reactions are all detrimental, but the good news is that the damage can be reduced to a tolerable level.

Nicotine produces cardiovascular effects that last for thirty to forty minutes after smoking such as increased heart rate, increased blood pressure, and decreased blood flow to the lungs and skin. A study conducted at Auburn University found that 400 milligrams of vitamin C normalized the effects of nicotine. This fact may be related to the action of nicotine that lowers blood levels of vitamin C.

Carbon monoxide binds so strongly to red blood cells that it renders them useless for carrying oxygen for prolonged periods. The best defense is to avoid the carbon dioxide of smoke, but short of that, the next best defense is to keep the rest of the blood cells healthy. Vitamin B-12, folic acid, iron, and zinc are important nutrients in the production of red blood cells. Vitamin E is critical to the lifespan of red blood cells—a vitamin E deficiency causes the red blood cells to rupture prematurely.

Vitamin C and the amino acid cysteine (L-cysteine) protect the arteries from reactions with aldehyde. Aldehyde can damage arterial linings in such a way as to initiate the plaque process referred to as "cholesterol deposits." Beta-carotene, Pycnogenol and selenium, the ever-so-important trace mineral, help protect the arteries from undesirable oxidation and free-radical attacks.

Supplements to Reduce the Cardiovascular Effects of Smoking

You may wish to consider the following food supplements to reduce the adverse effects of cigarette smoking on the heart and arteries. You may also wish to refer to Chapter 13, which deals with protection against lung cancer.

In the case of lung cancer the "alternative" strategy can produce results superior to the "prudent" strategy. However, in the case of cardiovascular effects and smoking, the alternative strategy only reduces the damage and is not as good as the prudent approach. But it is a thousand times better than not doing anything while you smoke. And as always, combining the prudent and alternative strategies is the ideal situation. Someday we will all be ideal! Keep trying to kick the habit.

TABLE 18.5
Supplements for Smokers

Nutrient	Daily Amount
Vitamin C	400–2,000 mg
Vitamin E	200–400 IU
L-cysteine	500–1,500 mg
Folic acid	400–800 mcg
Vitamin B-12	25–100 mcg
Zinc	15–25 mg
Selenium	100–200 mcg
Iron	10–25 mg

More Heart Help for Everyone

The nutrients discussed in this chapter help prevent heart attacks by keeping your blood free-flowing. The nutrients discussed in the next chapter will keep your heart strong and beating properly.

However, for those who may already be heart patients there are more stringent nutritional measures that you can consider. Chapter 20 will discuss a nutritional-medical combination approach that can make a big difference. If this applies to you, you may wish to consult with your nutrition-oriented physician to see if this adjunct therapy would be useful in your case.

19

A Strong Heartbeat and Heart Tonics

In addition to keeping the blood free-flowing through the arteries, we must keep the heart, a special muscle, healthy. In addition, the heartbeat must be kept regular. Certain nutrients specially energize the heart because the heart produces its energy differently than other muscles.

The heart cells rely on mitochondria for energy production, and that requires Coenzyme Q-10 (CoQ-10). The main energy comes from fat molecules, not the carbohydrate molecules normal muscles use. This requires an amino acid-like compound, L-carnitine.

The heartbeat itself depends on the minerals potassium, calcium, and magnesium for its regulation. Other nutrients are also involved in keeping a strong, regular beat.

Let's look at the roles of some critical nutrients in terms of heart health.

Coenzyme Q-10

The importance of Coenzyme Q-10 (CoQ-10) in slowing the aging process was discussed in Chapter 5. However, this nutrient is better known for its ability to strengthen hearts.

Our ability to make this important compound seems to decrease as we age. In some people the ability to make CoQ-10 becomes so impaired that they depend almost entirely on their diets for CoQ-10. In such cases CoQ-10 can be said to assume vitamin status. CoQ-10 can be found in many fresh foods, but it is a fragile compound that is easily destroyed by oxidation, processing, and cooking. Organ meats, spinach, whole grains, beef, sardines, peanuts, nuts, and seeds are good sources of CoQ-10 or its precursors.

CoQ-10 is a very popular food supplement in Japan and several other countries. It may become the nutrient of the 1990s in the U.S. once the research results are known. It is ironic that the nutrient is so popular elsewhere, because the two leading CoQ-10 researchers are Americans, Dr. Karl Folkers of the University of Texas and Dr. Emile Bliznakov of the Lupus Research Institute in Ridgefield, Connecticut. I had the pleasure of describing some of Dr. Folker's earlier research on CoQ-10 (it was known as ubiquinone then) in the original *Supernutrition* in 1975.

At the conclusion of a 1983 conference on CoQ-10 at the Max Planck Institute for Biochemistry in Martinsfried, Germany, where Nobel Prize and Priestley medal winners reported on their research with CoQ-10, Dr. Folkers made the following remarks.

"We have heard that patients in advanced cardiac failure, who had only a few months to live, under close medical care, have revealed almost miraculous improvement after treatment with CoQ-10, and such is a step of progress in cardiology.

"Proof of effectiveness of CoQ-10 in cardiology is now known to medical science. . . . Proof of the safety of CoQ-10 is known."

There are countless studies in the medical literature, but the general reader would probably rather read the excellent review of the research by Dr. Bliznakov and reporter Gerald Hunt in their book *The Miracle Nutrient: Coenzyme Q-10*.[1]

Gerald Hunt reported on one dramatic case in *Omni* magazine (1987): "The patient was in her early fifties. Because of rapidly degenerating heart function, doctors gave the woman no more than a couple of weeks to live. Today, two years later, she is alive and well, her heart is strong, and she is remarkably active."

The woman was in a CoQ-10 study conducted by the University of Bonn. Her heart output had dropped to life-threatening levels. Conventional medicines such as digitalis, beta-blockers, and vasodilators had no beneficial effect. Within five weeks of CoQ-10 supplementation her heart was pumping healthy amounts (4.5 liters per minute).

CoQ-10 is important to a strong heartbeat in two ways. First, it keeps the beat regular, and second, it keeps the heartbeat coordinated and strong. In 1981 Dr. Folkers noticed in patients on CoQ-10 that were being very closely monitored for two months that their arrhythmias disappeared or were greatly reduced.

Tyrosine

The amino acid tyrosine decreases the incidence of an extremely harmful heartbeat irregularity, ventricular fibrillation. Not all heartbeat irregularities (arrhythmias) are harmful. Some are just skipped beats due to stress or excitement and have no untoward consequences. However, ventricular fibrillation is to be avoided if possible.

Studies show that tyrosine is particularly effective in reducing the incidence of ventricular fibrillation.[2]

L-Carnitine

L-carnitine is an amino acid–like compound that does not enter into protein structures. Its purpose is to help muscle cells, especially heart cells, use fats for energy. L-carnitine helps carry fats into the mitochondria, the power plants of cells, and stimulates the oxidation of the fats to produce energy. L-carnitine is critical for a strong heart.

As people age they tend to produce less L-carnitine. Good diets may keep us adequately nourished in L-carnitine, but poor diets may produce a deficiency severe enough to impair the heart.

Inosine

Inosine is a nutritional nucleotide that helps the heart produce energy.[3] Inosine increases the production of the energy compound ATP in the heart.

Inosine helps normalize irregular heartbeats, according to research in Japan.[4]

Magnesium

Magnesium is a gatekeeper mineral that helps control the passage of calcium and potassium into and out of nerve and heart cells. The flow of calcium, sodium, and potassium in and out of cells generates electrical gradients. These gradients travel along nerve dendrites to "fire" the heartbeat.

The nerve impulse triggers the release of calcium in heart cells. Calcium inside the heart cells causes the contraction. Magnesium within the cells assists relaxation.

Magnesium is needed for heartbeat regularity. Low magnesium levels can cause severe arrhythmias (irregular heartbeats) of the ventricle of the heart resulting in sudden death. It has been found that injecting magnesium into the blood of heart attack victims upon their arrival at the hospital greatly reduces the chance of deadly arrhythmias.[5-7]

In a study at the Reggio Calabria University in Italy, patients who received magnesium for seven to ten days had their arrhythmias significantly reduced, including preventricular contractions, couplets, and ventricular tachycardia runs.[8]

People on diuretics (water pills) for high blood pressure run into a problem with potassium loss in the urine, but they also have a magnesium loss that is rarely recognized by physicians. Whenever one is advised to eat more bananas or oranges for potassium, he or she should also improve magnesium intake.

Potassium

Potassium, like magnesium, affects heart rhythm. The over-refined foods of today have removed much of the original potassium and replaced it with sodium. This problem has been amplified by the space program, which had to limit weight and bulk—even in astronauts' diets. Super-refined foods were used at first.

Apollo 15 lunar explorers David Scott and James Irwin both developed irregular heart rhythms due to potassium loss. They probably had a magnesium deficiency, too, but the medical profession hasn't yet tuned into magnesium.

NASA physician Dr. Charles Berry first noticed a few isolated premature heartbeats from James Irwin when he was working hard on the moon. At liftoff from the moon Astronaut Irwin had a series of ten irregular heartbeats. He suffered a series of arrhythmias during three hours of transferring moon rocks to the command module. David Scott's arrhythmias occurred just before splashdown. He had taken aspirin to ease a shoulder pain, which increased his potassium excretion.

Starting with Apollo 16, astronauts had potassium-enriched foods and snacks added to their diets, and they were placed on a potassium-loaded preflight diet. Potassium will be discussed more in Chapter 21 on blood pressure.

Taurine

As I said before, the amino acid taurine has been widely researched in Japan for its role in normalizing both blood pressure and blood cholesterol levels. Taurine also strengthens the heart.

Dr. J. Azuma demonstrated that taurine is effective in the treatment of congestive heart disease, even in cases where drugs were not helpful.[9] This has been confirmed by Dr. K. Takihara and colleagues.[10]

Vitamin E

The ability of the heart to beat is influenced by many factors. The heartbeat is controlled by an electrical center called the A-V node. Vitamin E is involved in intracellular calcium transport. In the case of heart rhythm, vitamin E deficiency decreases the myocardial resistance to cellular calcium excess, resulting in premature beats induced by calcium.[11] Several studies have shown that vitamin E restores normal heart rhythm.[12]

Bioflavonoids

Pycnogenol, a bioflavonoid, improves capillary permeability. This is also one of the many benefits of vitamin E, but bioflavonoids and vitamin E go about this task in different ways. Capillary permeability is not important to heart rhythm but is very important in keeping arteries healthy and preventing congestive heart failure.

Quercetin is a bioflavonoid found in onions, broccoli, and squash that is a potent anticancer nutrient and membrane stabilizer. Quercetin also reduces the production of harmful prostaglandins that lead to the blood-clotting leukotrienes.

Fish Oil

Australian researchers have discovered that fish oil (EPA) prevents ventricular fibrillation in laboratory animals.[13]

Dimethylglycine

Dr. Mitchell Pries found that dimethylglycine (DMG) helped heart patients in several ways. Volunteers taking DMG had fewer arrhythmias.

Supplements for a Strong Heart

You may wish to consider the following supplements for a strong heart. Don't forget to include copper, chromium, and silicon for strong arteries.

TABLE 19.1
Supplements for a Strong Heart

Nutrient	Daily Amount
CoQ-10	15–60 mg
L-carnitine	250–500 mg
Potassium	100–250 mg
Magnesium	300–600 mg
Copper	1–2 mg
Chromium	100–200 mcg
Taurine	250–3,000 mg
Bioflavonoids (quercetin, Pycnogenol)	250–1,000 mg
Inosine	500–1,000 mg
Dimethylglycine (DMG)	100–300 mg
Fish oil (EPA)	2–4 capsules

20

Nutritional Medicines for Heart Patients

The distinctions between nutrition and the use of nutrients as medicine are blurred by the inherent complexities and imposed legal definitions involved. However, one distinction is as sharp as a razor's edge—nutritional medicine is the domain of the physician and is not to be tinkered with unless the patient is under the continued guidance of a nutritionally oriented physician.

However, everyone should know what can be achieved with nutritional medicine so that all may request its benefits from their physicians. Although the nutrients described in this section are readily available without prescription, their use by a heart patient should be a part of the overall therapy and under the supervision of a physician.

Unfortunately, not every physician is aware of these new techniques, so you may have to educate such a physician with the references quoted, or seek out nutritionally oriented physicians from directories published by the International Academy of Preventive Medicine, the American Academy of Medical Preventics, *Prevention* magazine, your local health food store, or other sources.

Of course, physicians have also been misled by earlier studies with heart drugs. According to a study published in the November 11, 1989 issue of the *British Medical Journal*, the family of heart drugs called "calcium channel blockers" may not prevent a first heart attack or even reduce your chances of dying from a heart attack. Investigators analyzed data from twenty-eight controlled clinical trials involving over 19,000 heart patients being treated with five different calcium channel blockers including the widely prescribed Cardizam. No significant improvement in heart disease was found.

In March 1990 a study at Mount Sinai School of Medicine was the second to find that widely used drugs that are supposed to treat irregular heartbeats may actually increase the risk of sudden death in such people as congestive heart patients. The second study of procainamide, tocainide, and encainide found problems with each.

It's certain that we need to stress nutrition adjunct therapy regardless of what physicians may believe about the latest wonder heart drug. Sometimes time tells us more than the early drug-company tests do.

Soon all physicians will be aware of the exciting advances in nutrition adjunct therapy that are reported to drop the heart disease death rate to a small fraction of normal. The nutrients involved are a few minerals, enzymes, and mucopolysaccharides.

The first point that heart disease patients should know is that if you do suffer a heart attack, vitamins C and E, plus the trace mineral selenium, can limit the damage. As Dr. Joe McCord of the University of South Alabama College of Medicine stated in *American Health* (July/August 1986), "A full complement of vitamins C and E and selenium would be beneficial in withstanding the onslaught of a heart attack."

After a heart attack, when the blood starts flowing better and delivering oxygen to the oxygen-starved cells of the heart, tremendous amounts of free radicals are liberated. Antioxidant nutrients can quench many of the free radicals and prevent much tissue death (infarcted area).

Thus, it's not the actual blockage that is so damaging, but the reperfusion upon opening the coronaries back up.

In experiments with surgery-induced heart attacks in laboratory animals, antioxidants have helped the animals recover 68% of heart function compared to only 48% in the animals not receiving the antioxidants.

Fish oil (EPA) has also been shown to have a protective effect on the reperfusion.

Research by Dr. Hans Nieper of Hanover, West Germany brought about advances that cut the heart disease death rate by 95%. Dr. Nieper may be reached at his clinic at 21 Sedanstrasse, 3000 Hanover, Germany (phone 0511-31-11-11). Further advances by Dr. Lester Morrison of the Institute For Arteriosclerosis Research in Los Angeles may cut the death rate even further. Let's look at Dr. Nieper's findings first.

Dr. Nieper describes his nutritional-medical therapy as simple and remarkably effective. It can give years of extra life to heart patients—or anyone, for that matter. Dr. Nieper points out that one does not have to have heart disease to use the therapy, and he claims that there are absolutely no side effects.

Dr. Nieper's therapy involves treatment with oral supplements of magnesium, potassium, and an enzyme extracted from pineapple, bromelain. The enzyme acts as a "pipe cleaner," according to Dr. Nieper, to clean out the arteries.

In trials with more than 150 serious heart disease patients lasting over two years, Dr. Nieper found the therapy to be 95% effective. Without the therapy 24% to 30% of the patients (36–45 persons) would have been expected to die from heart attacks over the two-year test period.

Dr. Gerhard Schuurmann of Bergsteinfurt, West Germany has repeated Dr. Nieper's therapy with 150 of his own patients and has found even better results. At this writing he reports that not a single patient has had a heart attack since undergoing the therapy.

Dr. Gary Gordon (then of Sacramento in private practice, now the medical director of a firm in Hayward) used the nutritional therapy and found that over 85% of his 700 heart patients got dramatic relief of symptoms. Less than 1% suffered a fatal attack during the two-year test by Dr. Gordon.

Published results from Dr. Lester Morrison's studies at the Institute For Arteriosclerosis Research show that cerebral, coronary, and peripheral vascular circulation significantly improved in about 75% of the patients improving their life-style, reducing dietary fat, and taking the following food supplements:

- phosphatidyl cholines (from soy beans)
- mucopolysaccharides (MPS) [also called glyco-saminoglycans] (from sea plant or trachea extracts)
- elastomucoprotease enzyme inhibitors (bovine aorta extracts)

Dr. Morrison has found that the MPS help maintain blood vessel elasticity and maintain blood slipperiness, as do the phosphatidyl cholines, while reducing blood LDL cholesterol and triglycerides. Dr. Morrison made the elastomucoprotease enzyme inhibitors a part of his program based on his observation that they demonstrate anticlotting properties as measured by a procedure called the Chandler loop procedure.

The group of similar food factors called MPS complex include fairly common compounds such as heparin, chondroitin sulfate A, and hyaluronic acid.

Dr. Morrison has found that these food factors were strikingly effective in the reduction of death rate, the morbidity rate, and the complication rate from coronary heart disease, cerebrovascular disease (stroke), and peripherovascular disease. The food factors had distinctive cholesterol- and triglyceride-lowering effects with emphasis on the reduction of the harmful LDL cholesterol and the increase of the protective HDL cholesterol. There were no toxic or side effects reported in the studies. To be effective, they must be taken as food concentrates rather than as the whole food.

Dr. Morrison also recommends bromelain and silicon.

Silicon

Silicon is essential for artery health. Silicon was discussed in Chapter 10 on osteoporosis in regard to being "the glue that holds bone tissue together." Silicon is also the glue that holds arteries together. Silicon and MPS are very important to artery structural integrity, elasticity, and permeability.

Silicon may also be involved in the transport of fats from artery walls and in binding to bile.

Silicon is a component of many dietary fibers and may help explain some of the benefits of soluble fiber. Because of our refined low-fiber diets we tend to lose body silicon reserves as we age.

Autopsies have shown that silicon, like chromium, is present in the arteries of persons free of heart disease in much greater quantities than in the arteries of those dying from heart disease.

Bromelain was described in Chapter 18.

If you wish to advise your physician of this research, you will find references 1–8 helpful.

Aspirin

You may also wish to keep an eye on the ongoing aspirin studies. The results of the Veterans Administration Cooperative Study showed that aspirin has a protective effect against acute myocardial infarction (heart attack) in men with unstable angina, and the data indicate a similar effect on mortality.[9]

It was good news! Around the world people pricked up their ears to listen more closely to the evening news as they were informed that aspirin might help reduce their risk of heart attacks. No dieting, no worrying about dietary cholesterol or fats, no balancing the diet for better nutrition, no exercising—just include an aspirin a day to keep the cardiologist away. Could it be that simple?

Aspirin is a drug with a few side effects that can even be fatal on occasion—and it can be a deadly poison when overdosed.

The clinical study that indicates that aspirin may reduce heart attacks by almost half was a well-designed clinical trial. A larger number of participants would make the study more meaningful, but there is enough good data there to suggest that the effect of aspirin should be expected to reduce heart attacks by at least 30%. The day after this study was published in the *New England Journal of Medicine*[10] a similar study was published in the *British Medical Journal* that concluded that aspirin had no effect on heart attacks.

The problem with the British study is that it included only 5,139 subjects, whereas the American study included 22,071. There were too few heart attack victims in the smaller study to allow any difference in frequency to be demonstrated with statistical significance.

The aspirin study was not a real surprise. Earlier studies had demonstrated that aspirin reduced the risk of having a second heart attack in men who had been hospitalized with their first heart attack. The newer study confirmed that aspirin worked in healthy men as well. Aspirin works via reducing the tendency for blood to clot in the coronary arteries.

Several researchers have noted another very important difference. The English study used plain aspirin while the American study used aspirin buffered with magnesium. They feel that the amount of magnesium was significant to persons severely deficient in magnesium. The importance of this question remains to be resolved.

No quantities are discussed here because of the great variation in individual responses, which necessitates monitoring by a physician.

Dimethylglycine (DMG)

Dimethylglycine has been found to help heart patients having angina pectoris. DMG has an oxygen-sparing effect because it aids cells in extracting energy from food via ATP production in a manner that uses less oxygen. DMG also improves circulation and cardiac output as well as normalizing blood pressure and heart rhythm.

The research of Dr. Mitchell Pries was discussed in Chapter 17. In clinical evaluations by Dr. Pries of over 400 geriatric cardiovascular patients, there was major improvement in the following areas with DMG:

1. increase in feeling of well-being, vitality, and mobility
2. improvement in circulatory insufficiency
3. decrease in high blood cholesterol
4. reduction in angina pain

5. fewer irregular heartbeats
6. decrease of high blood pressure
7. improvement in heart response to stress tests

After mentioning the benefits of DMG (then known as its conjugate with calcium gluconate and called calcium pangamate) in *Supernutrition for Healthy Hearts* I received hundreds of letters and even had heart patients who were formerly incapacitated drive to my house from states far away to show me their outstanding progress and to thank me personally. This is why I write to share my research.

Supplements for Heart Patients

Heart patients should optimize their nutrition along the lines presented earlier in this chapter and in the preceding chapter, plus they should consider the following additional nutritional adjuncts. Keep in mind that heart patients should most certainly inform their physicians of their supplement program so that they may be properly monitored. You must work with your physician as a partner in health. It does no one any good to keep secrets from his or her physician. You should also

---

TABLE 20.1
Supplements for Heart Patients

Nutrient	Daily Amount
Mucopolysaccharides (MPS)	250–1,000 mg
Dimethylglycine (DMG)	100–500 mg
Silicon	10–50 mg
Bromelain	500–1,000 mg
Vitamin E	400–1,000 mg
Potassium	100–500 mg
Magnesium	250–500 mg
Bioflavonoids (including quercetin and Pycnogenol)	500–1,000 mg
Coenzyme Q-10 (CoQ-10)	30–60 mg
(Aspirin)	(under direction of physician)

---

check with your health care professionals about a walking regimen and your exercise program.

As I advised in the prevention section, the food supplements discussed here offer protection from high-fat, high-cholesterol, and low-fiber diets for the heart patient. But keep in mind that high-fat, low-fiber diets may be linked to bowel cancer. Chapter 14 discussed protection from bowel cancer.

21

Normalizing Blood Pressure

—————————————— ■ ——————————————

If your blood pressure is normal or low, you can skip this chapter. If your systolic (top number) is above 130 or your diastolic (bottom number) is above 85, it is in your best interest to read on. Elevated blood pressure is indeed life-shortening. Fortunately, high blood pressure is easy to correct even if you insist on eating a salt-laden diet.

You should know your blood pressure. It should be taken monthly if normal and weekly if controlled by drugs or dietary measures. You should take daily measurements while you are determining whether or not you are salt-sensitive, and also while you are making changes to normalize your blood pressure.

Your Blood Pressure

Now before you start with the excuses—you don't have time or a place to go to have your blood pressure taken—consider that one of the best investments that you can make in your health is to buy one of the new inexpensive automatic sphyg-momanometers (blood pressure measuring devices). They are completely automatic and accurate and cost about the same as two or three tanks of gasoline.

It puzzles me why everyone has a bathroom scale when they can see if they're putting on weight by looking in the mirror and feel if they are by how snugly their clothes fit, and yet most of these same people won't buy a personal sphygmomanometer, which is more critical to their health and costs no more than the scale. Both instruments can be purchased with automatic features that directly register the result with little operator skill required.

Table 21.1 shows how important blood pressure is. If you don't monitor your blood pressure regularly, then you won't know that corrective action should be taken to preserve your normal life span.

Frequent blood pressure measurement also helps you detect unsuspected fluctuations that may be linked to life-style or emotions. If you can identify such blood pressure–raising events, you can learn to normalize your blood pressure without the need for drugs or dietary manipulation.

TABLE 21.1
Blood Pressure and Life Expectancy

| Age | | Blood Pressure | Added Life Expectancy (years) | |
Men	Women		Men	Women
35		120/80	41.5	?
		130/90	37.5	?
		140/95	32.5	?
		150/100	25	?
45		120/80	32	37
		130/90	29	35.5
		140/95	26	32
		150/100	20.5	28.5
55		120/80	23.5	27.5
		130/90	22.5	27
		140/95	19.5	24.5
		150/100	17.5	23.5

(Courtesy Metropolitan Life Insurance Company)

Salt Is Not the Problem

We hear so much about cutting back on salt. "We eat too much salt." How do they know I eat too much salt? Perhaps I am eating so little salt that cutting back may cause an electrolyte deficiency in me. Okay, my point is that general advice for populations may not apply to the individual but may rather be harmful to the individual.

My second point is that not many people are affected by reasonable changes in dietary salt. All this talk about salt and blood pressure, and yet only about eight percent of the population will experience either an increase or decrease in blood pressure in response to a similar change in salt intake.

Using an intravenous infusion of salt Dr. Myron Weinberger of Indiana University determined that about one fourth of those with normal blood pressure are salt-sensitive, and about one half of those with high blood pressure are salt-sensitive.

Dr. Weinberger also determined that sensitivity to salt seems to increase as people get older. However, this was a cross-sectional study, not a longitudinal study. The same individuals will have to be followed over a long period of time to establish if this is a fact.

However, if people do tend to develop salt sensitivity as they age, it would then have to be determined if this was due to prolonged mineral imbalance or if it was a function of the aging process.

A later study by Dr. Judy Miller and her colleagues, also at Indiana University, used the salt-infusion method to find that those sensitive to salt usually had an abnormal amount of a protein called haptoglobin in their blood. This was linked to genes acquired from their parents. If both parents had this genetic defect, the children were very likely to be salt-sensitive, too.[1]

Also, a preliminary study shows that sodium can affect the arteries' dilation and constriction even if the effect isn't strong enough to affect blood pressure. Older subjects placed on a low-salt diet for four days regained the ability to dilate as much as younger persons. Drs. Ross Feldman and Christine Sinkey of the University of Iowa believe that low-salt diets can stave off age-associated malfunctions in artery receptors that control dilation.

A geneticist at Indiana University, Dr. Judy Miller, has developed a simple blood test that identifies those who are salt-sensitive and most likely to benefit from a low-salt diet. The genes that regulate haptoglobin-1 are the same genes that determine salt-sensitivity, according to Dr. Miller.

My third point is that salt is a minor part of the picture. The main concern should be potassium and potassium-to-sodium ratio. When potassium intake is adequate the blood pressures of even salt-sensitive persons are not affected by salt loading.

Modern diets contain so much salt that it's hard to believe that salt was once a luxury as well as a dietary essential. In fact, salt was so scarce that it was once used as payment for goods and services. The term "salary" is said to be derived from this practice, as well as the phrase "not worth his salt." The esteem held for salt is especially noticed in the Bible. As an example, "Ye are the salt of the earth."[2]

The problem is that since salt has been so scarce down through the history of man until recent times, man has adapted to low-salt diets by being efficient in retaining salt. The daily amount of salt that we need is probably around 200–400 milligrams, yet the average American is getting twenty times that much.

Salt is chemically called sodium chloride. Sodium and potassium are two minerals that are in a tug-of-war with each other in the body. Potassium is used primarily inside the cells, and sodium is primarily used in fluids surrounding the cells. Optimal body chemistry requires a balance between the two, which is chiefly regulated by the sodium regulatory mechanism. However, about 20% of the population cannot maintain optimal sodium and potassium balance when they eat a high-salt diet. The salt load combined with their strong retention of sodium is too great a strain on their regulatory system.

Thus, in certain people, dietary salt above a certain level has been shown to increase blood pressure. And it has been shown that if these same persons are put on a diet that contains less than that very low level of salt, their blood pressure level will move toward normal. It has also been shown that an equal percentage of the population will respond to this same very-low-salt diet with a rise in blood pressure. Again the old saw that one man's meat (or diet) is another man's poison.

It is interesting to note that the vast majority of us are not very sensitive to salt in terms of blood pressure. Why should the majority have to succumb to a low-salt diet or be lectured about eating less salt when in truth it has no effect on their blood pressure? Or more important, why should someone who will react to a low-salt diet with an increase in blood pressure take the risk of following the popular advice to eat a low-salt diet?

It does seem prudent for salt-sensitive persons to avoid salt, but these people do not respond to a cutback in salt until the salt content dips below a level that is virtually impossible to achieve with conventional processed foods. Only a natural diet of unprocessed foods seems to offer a potassium-to-sodium ratio that will enable these genetically impaired individuals to normalize their blood pressure by salt restriction alone. Therefore, the prudent advice seems to be of little practical value. Drugs do help these individuals whether or not they cut back on salt, but greatest success is obtained with the lowest drug doses and a good potassium-to-sodium-ratio diet.

There is no nutritional virtue in eating a high-salt diet, but if we have too many groundless dietary restrictions intended as good advice for the masses, they end up being counterproductive for the individual. The real risk factor is high blood pressure, not salt content of the diet.

We should all determine if we are salt-sensitive or not. I am not salt-sensitive. I have known this for years by observation of salt intake compared to blood pressure. I have gone on high-salt diets. In addition, I added sweets to my experimental high-salt diets, because most salt-sensitive people are especially sensitive to the combination of sugar and salt. This phenomenon was first discovered with laboratory rats and then confirmed in people. Personally, I am not salt-sensitive in terms of near-term influence on blood pressure, but I know others who say they eat a potato chip and retain water.

Salt is an indirect cause of elevated blood pressure in those individuals so affected. The direct cause of high blood pressure may be deficiencies of the minerals potassium, magnesium, and calcium and the vitamins A and C, according to researchers at the Oregon Health Sciences University in Portland.[3] The study of data from 10,372 persons indicated that calcium was the nutrient for which reduced intake was most consistent in hypertensive individuals. Those with the highest salt consumption had the fewest cases of high blood pressure.

Of course, if your physician has placed you on a low-salt diet, you should follow your physician's advice. However, there is no need for the masses to go on a low-salt diet without a specific indication that it would be beneficial or desirable. If you enjoy a low-salt diet, that is something else—but be sure that you are not one of the few who have increased blood pressure on low-salt diets.

The genetically impaired individuals who experience elevated blood pressure on today's salty diets can be helped by adding more potassium to the diet. Where do they get the potassium from if they won't shift to the more natural (but less tasty) diets that fed man through the ages? They can consider using a salt substitute, which is potassium chloride instead of sodium chloride, that almost identically improves the flavor of foods.

Potassium

The importance of potassium to normal blood pressure was demonstrated in clinical trials in the 1930s, laboratory animals in 1957, and population studies in Japan in 1959.[4] More recent confirmations have come from a 1987 University of California study[5] and another Japanese study,[6] an Australian study,[7] and an English study.[8]

However, just as is the case with salt, it may be that not all individuals respond equally well to potassium. My experience, however, has been that when someone doesn't respond to potassium, he or she is also magnesium-deficient and needs both magnesium and potassium supplementation.

Potassium encourages the body to excrete sodium and water. Potassium also helps keep the artery wall thickness normal and make the artery walls more flexible.[9]

Potassium and sodium help move nutrients into cells and

waste products out of cells by an osmotic system called the sodium-potassium pump. Many nutrients are dragged along with the ions (due to charge attraction) as the ions are pumped across the membrane. A potassium deficiency results in a tired feeling that can lead to general weakness.

The body uses energy provided by a molecule called ATP to move potassium into a cell and sodium out of the cell. Nearly a third of the calories we eat are used to provide energy to run the countless sodium-potassium pumps in cell membranes. Thus, in healthy, well-nourished persons, sodium tends to be present in higher concentrations near the outside membrane surface, and potassium tends to be in higher concentration inside the cell.

The sodium-potassium pump is energized by food metabolism, but there is another pump that gets its energy directly from the sodium-potassium pump. This is the calcium pump. The calcium pump's function is to keep the amount of calcium inside a cell many thousands of times lower than the external circulating calcium.

Calcium causes muscle cells to contract. When calcium is driven into a muscle cell, contraction results. This causes the heartbeat and constricts the walls of arteries. You can now see the delicate relationship between sodium, potassium, and calcium. As they are all involved in a proper heartbeat and rhythm, they are also involved in controlling blood pressure.

An excellent book that helps you select foods based on their ratio of potassium to sodium is *The K Factor*.[10] Anyone with high blood pressure should read this book. The name comes from the chemical symbol for potassium (kalium), K.

A banana or a glass of orange juice a day can go a long way toward providing the potassium you need. Apple and grapefruit juices also have good potassium-to-sodium ratios. Of course, replacing highly processed foods with natural whole foods will be a major help in correcting the potassium-to-sodium balance. But don't forget that magnesium is needed as well.

Vitamin C

In May 1990 at the annual meeting of the American Society for Clinical Nutrition, two studies reported that persons with high vitamin C intakes had significantly lower blood pressure than those with low vitamin C intakes. The first study was conducted by Drs. Leslie Cohen and Elaine Feldman of the Medical College of Georgia, while the second study was reported by Dr. Elaine Choi of Tufts University.

At the same meeting Dr. David Trout of the USDA's Beltsville Human Nutrition Research Center reported that in a study of twelve persons with borderline hypertension, a daily one-gram vitamin C supplement reduced systolic blood pressure.

Calcium

Many of us have appreciated for many years the roles of calcium, magnesium, and selenium in maintaining normal blood pressures, but it wasn't until 1984 that the scientific community was startled by the observation that calcium intake may be even more important to maintaining normal blood pressure than avoiding sodium. Dr. David McCarron of the Oregon Health Sciences University published his analysis of the dietary intakes of 10,372 adults. He concluded that of the seventeen nutrients examined, calcium was most consistently associated with blood pressure.

His research group also found that people with high blood pressure also tended to have lower intakes of potassium, sodium, and vitamins A and C. Hypertensives had lower intakes of dairy products than of any other food group. Their most startling comment to the establishment nutritionists was that nutritional deficiencies, rather than excesses, distinguished subjects with high blood pressure from those with normal blood pressure.[3] Now where have I heard that before?

In the same month Dr. McCarron's group published two articles in *Nutrition Reviews* with the same message.[11,12] The establishment tried to explain the results away, but they had to take notice.

The following year a research group at the University of Wisconsin confirmed the effect. They monitored the dietary calcium intake in eighty-one normotensive and thirty-four hypertensive women aged thirty-five to sixty-five years. Then they gave supplements providing one and a half grams of calcium daily to half the women in each group for four years. The calcium had no effect on blood pressure in the women with normal blood pressure, but those with high blood pressure had significantly lowered systolic pressure (the first number).[13]

Also in 1985, an interesting study in the Netherlands showed that excess dietary sodium increased the amount of calcium and potassium excreted. The study confirmed that men with higher calcium intakes had lower systolic blood pressure than those consuming less calcium. The scientists concluded that sodium intake may have an influence on blood pressure through its effects on urinary calcium and potassium excretion, and that these effects may be more pronounced in people with a low calcium intake.[14,15] Of all the research done on blood pressure in the last twenty-five years, this may be one of the most significant studies. How many physicians do you think know about it?

In another study from Erasmus University in the Netherlands in 1986 it was found that 1,000 milligrams a day of a calcium supplement significantly lowered the diastolic pressure (the second number).[16]

In 1986 a Wayne State University group looked at the relationship in another way. They fed hypertensive subjects and salt-sensitive subjects diets containing either 360 or 930 milligrams of calcium with either 1,000 or 4,000 milligrams of sodium in the daily diet. They found that a high-sodium diet combined with low calcium intake caused systolic blood pressures to rise in both normotensives and hypertensives. This sodium-induced effect on blood pressure was partially to completely reversed when calcium intake was increased. The addition of calcium to the high-sodium diet caused an increase in both the urinary excretion of sodium and the blood level of renin, the kidney enzyme that affects the hormone angiotensin, which in turn influences blood-vessel constriction and thus blood pressure.[17]

They also found that calcium added to a low-sodium diet increased the urinary excretion of sodium but did not affect blood renin activity. The researchers concluded that the normalization of blood pressure by calcium is a result of calcium-induced loss of sodium in the urine and blockage of sodium-induced expansion of blood volume, as indicated by the increase in blood renin activity.

Thus we have found that calcium increases sodium excretion and that sodium increases calcium excretion. What needs to be studied further is the total synergistic interrelationship between calcium, magnesium, potassium, and sodium.

Magnesium

Magnesium is also involved in the retention of potassium in the cells. Next to potassium, magnesium is the predominant cation in cells. One of its major roles is to help maintain the proper electrical charge gradient across cellular membranes. Magnesium also serves as a gatekeeper that slows the unwanted leakage of calcium back into cells.

Laboratory animal studies have shown that magnesium deficiency causes high blood pressure, and that increasing levels of dietary magnesium produce decreasing blood pressure.[18] Dr. Burton Altura feels that magnesium is one of the "most promising and least-used minerals when it comes to blood pressure control."

Researchers who studied sixty-one variables in the diets of healthy older men found that magnesium was most strongly linked to controlling blood pressure.[19] A high magnesium intake usually produces lower blood pressure.

A Hungarian study found that a daily magnesium supplement of 80 to 160 milligrams resulted in a decreased blood pressure.[20] A Swedish study found that a daily magnesium supplement equivalent to the RDA reduced both systolic and diastolic blood pressure. In Finland, when a magnesium-fortified table salt was used instead of regular table salt, blood pressures dropped.

Selenium

In 1965 Dr. K. O. Godwin found that animals fed low-selenium diets developed high blood pressure and electrocardiogram disturbances. The kidneys of persons having high blood pressure are usually lower than those in healthy persons.[21]

Selenium normalizes blood pressure by controlling prostaglandin production. Prostaglandins are hormonelike compounds that control many body functions. Dr. J. E. Vincent of Erasmus University (Rotterdam, Netherlands) found that selenium deficiency affected the production of prostaglandin A-2.

Selenium also helps the body tie up cadmium so that it doesn't do damage such as raising blood pressure.

Copper

Copper deficiency raises blood pressure. Persons with high blood pressure should ensure that they are not copper-deficient. The 1989 RDA range for copper is 1.5 to 3 milligrams per day. Most persons fall short of this range. Taking supplements of one to two milligrams of copper daily should ensure that further deficiency doesn't occur.

A study at the USDA Human Nutrition Research Center in Grand Forks, North Dakota have found that a combination of copper deficiency and stress had a 15% increase in systolic blood pressure. Those either copper-deficient or subjected to stress alone had much smaller increases in blood pressure.[22]

Coenzyme Q-10

Both clinical and animal studies have shown that Coenzyme Q-10 (CoQ-10) lowers high diastolic and systolic pressures.[23] Just as important, studies by some of these same researchers show that CoQ-10 has no effect on the blood pressure of those with normal blood pressure.[24]

Dr. Toru Yamagami has published four studies of CoQ-10 and blood pressure regulation.[25] He believes that CoQ-10 increases cell function so that arteries can both constrict and relax more efficiently. CoQ-10 has been discussed in several chapters in this book, especially Chapter 5 on aging and Chapter 20 on heart strength.

Taurine

The Japanese Stroke Prevention Center has found that dietary taurine lowers elevated blood pressure after four weeks of use.[26]

Fish Oil

High blood pressure is called a silent killer because it produces no pain or symptoms, yet it is a major risk factor for stroke and other diseases of the arteries. The good news is that fish oils—at least some of them—help normalize blood pressure.

Physicians at the Central Institute for Cardiovascular Research in the German Democratic Republic reported in July 1985 that a mackerel diet containing 2.2 grams of EPA daily produced a significantly lower systolic (upper number) blood pressure in eight of eight patients having an inherited disorder that produces abnormally high blood triglyceride and cholesterol levels and premature heart disease. The disease is called familial hyperlipoproteinemia. The mackerel diet also reduced blood cholesterol and triglycerides for a period of three months, after which they tended to drift back toward their previous values, as is the usual case with these patients and dietary modification.[27]

Later this research group studied fourteen patients having moderately high blood pressure (essential hypertension). The mackerel diet decreased systolic blood pressure by almost

10%. Whenever the subjects were returned to their normal diets their blood pressure increased again. When they were again given the mackerel diet their blood pressure dropped toward normal.

Other blood parameters associated with high blood pressure were also improved. Blood sodium (salt) levels decreased, and renin (a hormone produced in the kidney that greatly affects blood pressure) activity increased by 64%. The researchers concluded that these data suggest a beneficial effect of a mackerel diet on the cardiovascular risk in patients with mild essential hypertension.[28]

In 1986 researchers at the London Chest Hospital studied sixteen patients having mild hypertension. They were given MaxEPA fish oil capsules for twelve weeks in a placebo-controlled crossover study. Their blood pressure averaged 160/94 at the start of the study. After being on a placebo for six weeks their blood pressures remained at an average of 161/94.5, as would be expected. However, after being switched to MaxEPA fish oil capsules for six weeks their blood pressures dropped to an average of 151/92.5. The drop in systolic pressure was statistically significant.

Most patients reported that they preferred the fish oil supplements to their previous treatment. The researchers concluded that fish oil supplementation may provide a safe, more acceptable treatment for patients with mild essential systolic hypertension who are reluctant to embark on drug therapies.[29]

In 1989 Drs. Howard Knapp and Garret FitzGerald of Vanderbilt University confirmed that high doses of fish oil reduced high blood pressure in men.[30] Fifty milliliters per day of fish oil lowered the systolic pressure by an average of seven points (mmHg).

Because of biochemical individuality fish oils produce varying results. A summary of the general trends is given in Table 21.2.

TABLE 21.2
Summary of the effects of fish oil consumption on parameters related to heart disease

Parameter	Effect
Blood triglyceride level	Decrease (usually significant)
Blood cholesterol level	Decrease (inconsistent)
Blood HDL level	Tend to increase
Blood LDL level	Tend to decrease, but variable
Blood VLDL level	Decrease
Blood pressure	Usually decrease
Platelet aggregability	Decrease
Blood prostacyclin	Slight decrease
Platelet thromboxane	Decrease
Platelet number	Tend to decrease
Bleeding time	Increase
Blood linoleic level	Tend to decrease
Blood arachidonic acid level	Decrease
Blood EPA level	Increase
Blood DHA level	Increase
Platelet arachidonic acid	Decrease
Platelet Omega-3 fatty acids	Increase

Adapted from *Nutrition Today* (Nov/Dec 1986), p. 13.

Garlic

Regular use of garlic can lower high blood pressure by 12 to 30 points (mmHg) systolic and 7 to 20 (mmHg) diastolic. The mechanism through which garlic lowers high blood pressure is not known, but it is believed to involve prostaglandin regulation.[31]

Dimethylglycine (DMG)

A clinical study of fourteen hypertensive patients by Dr. Mitchell Pries showed an average reduction of 14 points

(mmHg) in diastolic pressure with 100 milligrams per day of DMG. The patients were also placed on a low-salt, modified-fat diet, and it is not clear how much of the reduction can be attributed to the diet change alone.

Supplements

The "alternative" strategy is first to determine if you are salt-sensitive, and to monitor your blood pressure to note behavioral or emotional influences. Then you help the body achieve potassium/sodium balance by increasing the amounts of other minerals that affect sodium regulation or normalize blood pressure via other normal regulatory channels.

In addition, the use of proper drugs is important. Your physician will determine which drug is best suited for you and monitor its progress. If the drug produces any side effects, all you have to do is inform your physician, and an alternative drug will be used.

As your diet and life-style improve your physician can cut back on your medication until, with luck, you can be completely weaned from it.

Minerals that help normalize blood pressure are calcium, magnesium, and selenium. Vitamins A, C, and E help most people, as do relaxation, weight normalization, and exercise. You don't have to take all of these supplements to gain control of your blood pressure. Different people will respond to different supplements depending upon the cause of their hypertension, their existing diet, and their biochemical individuality. The amounts of these supplements that have been effective are indicated in Table 21.3.

So the next time someone spouts the general advice to eat less salt, just keep your blood pressure down and realize that that person hasn't studied the original scientific literature in detail. One man's meat is another's poison, and the same can be said for the salted french-fried potatoes.

You can also consider normalizing your weight, exercising, giving up smoking, and avoiding unnecessary supersalted snacks to see if any of these alternatives are beneficial to you.

Not every incidence of high blood pressure can be normalized completely by diet. Sometimes there is organic or structural damage to the kidneys or adrenals that causes the problem—but even then, diet helps. Fruits and vegetables are rich in the minerals needed to maintain normal blood pressure. This is one reason that vegetarians have good blood pressures. But you don't have to be a vegetarian to take advantage of good mineral nutrition.

TABLE 21.3
Supplements for Normalizing Blood Pressure

Nutrient	Daily Amount
Potassium	50–200 mg
Try bananas and orange juice first, then supplements if more is needed.	
Calcium (taken in evening)	500–1,000 mg
Magnesium (taken in morning)	300–600 mg
Selenium	50–100 mcg
Vitamin A	5,000–10,000 IU
Vitamin C	250–1,000 mg
Vitamin E	200–400 IU
Fish oil	8–50 ml
Garlic	1–3 capsules

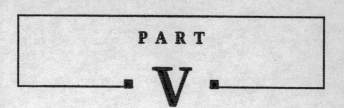

PART

V

Supernutrition Against Other Non-Germ Diseases

22

Arthritis

In the United States, the arthritis foundations and the Food and Drug Administration have for years labeled any mention of dietary relief for arthritis patients as quackery. This is not so in most countries. Now the U.S. "experts" will have to change their approach or be laughed at by the scientific community as well as the general population.

Too much evidence has accumulated over the past two decades to dismiss the correlation. There are two ways in which nutrition affects at least some arthritis patients. First, nutrients may alter immune and inflammatory responses so as to affect manifestations of arthritis. Second, food antigens can provoke sensitivity responses that result in rheumatologic symptoms.

An example of the first relationship is brought to mind by Dale Alexander. Dale Alexander appeared on countless radio shows telling the audience how many people have found relief from arthritis by taking cod-liver oil. He was called the "Cod-father." He described his experience in his book *Arthritis and Common Sense*. Now dozens of U.S. university laboratories are testing fish oil against arthritis. Fish oil contains EPA, which makes body compounds that control inflammation and pain. Dale Alexander didn't know about EPA, but he knew that cod-liver oil helped thousands of arthritis sufferers.

An example of the second relationship that comes to mind is the advice of Dr. Carlton Fredericks. He taught that the nightshade family of foods could sensitize some people so as to cause arthritis. Studies confirmed food sensitivities cause about 5% of arthritis and aggravate symptoms in about 30% of arthritis patients where they are not directly the cause.[1] But the experts continue to deny any association between diet and arthritis. Now we have these and newer nutrient-arthritis links to work with.

Arthritis is not one disease but several diseases possibly having several causes. The word "arthritis" is derived from the Greek word meaning joint and actually means "inflammation of the joint." There is little agreement on the causes of arthritis, but there is agreement on what is happening in the body that leads to the damage. Even though we may not know any or all of the events that start the disease process, we can interrupt the disease process and control arthritis.

Osteoarthritis is the most common form of arthritis. It involves the breakdown of cartilage, which eventually leads to damaged bone. It progresses fairly slowly and may be caused by the stress of wear and tear or even an infectious agent such as a bacterium. Nutritional deficiencies can aggravate the problem.

Rheumatoid arthritis is also an ailment that produces swollen and stiff joints, but it is more seasonal in nature, often beginning or worsening in colder weather. Rheumatoid arthritis begins as an inflammation in the synovial membrane that produces the fluid that lubricates bone joints. The cause of the inflammation is not known for certain, but many scientists feel that the body's immune system mistakenly attacks the joints. Diet and stress have also been suggested as being responsible for initiating the inflammation.

When the synovial membrane becomes inflamed the blood supply to the membrane increases, white blood cells gather in the membrane, and swelling occurs. The swelling can push the bone joints apart. The inflammation causes the synovial membrane to release chemicals called lysosomal enzymes that destroy cartilage and bone. The body tries to repair this damage but usually is successful only so far as to produce irregular patches and rough bumps. These outgrowths aggravate the problem and decrease joint function.

The disease process involves the inflammation and pain brought about by free radicals and certain undesirable prostaglandins. Free radicals were discussed in several earlier chapters (see Chapters 5 and 6). You don't have to review these nasty critters; just understand that free radical damage can be checked by nutritional antioxidants, and the undesirable prostaglandins can be balanced with desirable prostaglandins. The result is relief of pain and swelling due to arthritis.

The undesirable prostaglandins are members of the prostaglandin 2 family, which is derived from the polyunsaturated fat arachidonic acid. The desirable prostaglandins are members of the prostaglandin 1 family, which is derived from the polyunsaturated fats, cis-linoleic acid (CLA) and gamma-linolenic acid (GLA).

A very desirable member of the prostaglandin 1 family is prostaglandin E-1. Prostaglandin E-1 is necessary for normal function of the T-cells of the immune system (these cells reject foreign bodies). Prostaglandin E-1 reduces the release of inflammation-causing lysosomes and slows the formation of inflammation-producing prostaglandin E-2 by blocking the release of arachidonic acid from its storage sites.

It is becoming increasingly clear that there is an interrelationship between prostaglandins, vitamin E, aspirin, and steroid drugs. This interrelationship is too complex to discuss here, but it involves the biochemical pathways between the precursors, prostaglandins, and related compounds called leukotrienes.

Leukotrienes do have a positive function during wound healing, but under other conditions they are bothersome. Leukotrienes also produce inflammation, pain, and breast lumps in women called cystic mastitis. Vitamin E reduces leukotriene production by slowing the release of arachidonic acid from storage or by slowing the conversion of arachidonic acid to leukotrienes, according to Dr. David Cornwell of Ohio State University. Steroids act in a similar fashion.

Aspirin reduces the formation of prostaglandin E-2 and leukotrienes. This for the first time explains how aspirin can relieve pain and fever.

Rheumatology News reports that prostaglandin E-1 has

powerful healing effects on rheumatoid arthritis patients. As we will see later, this prostaglandin can be produced in our bodies provided we are adequately nourished with the proper raw materials.[2]

The proper balance of prostaglandins is achieved by balancing the dietary raw materials of the various prostaglandins. This is best achieved by adding the deficient polyunsaturates to balance the predominant polyunsaturate, arachidonic acid. This is accomplished by supplementing the diet with gamma-linolenic acid (GLA) and eicosapentaenoic acid (EPA). A popular food source of GLA is evening primrose oil, and an equally popular food source of EPA is fish oil.

Fish Oils (EPA)

Heart disease is what aroused scientific interest in fish oils, but now that we are beginning to understand the biochemistry involved we are seeing that EPA can bring benefit to a host of health problems.

Animal studies at Harvard indicated that EPA helps protect the body against attack by its own immune system in autoimmune diseases such as rheumatoid arthritis and lupus erythematosus.[3,4]

The researchers were studying the effects of EPA on the inflammatory process and kidney disease. They reasoned that if EPA reduces the body's production of inflammatory compounds, then it would aid arthritis and lupus sufferers. A key factor in the inflammation process is leukotriene B4 (LTB4). LTB4 can make a major contribution to joint discomfort and pain. Tissues can make LTB4 out of omega-6 fatty acids, but when omega-3 fatty acid EPA is present leukotriene B5 (LTB5) is made instead. LTB5 is relatively benign in comparison to LTB4.

A 1985 article in *Clinical Research* reported that fish oil supplements significantly improved rheumatoid arthritis patients. Dr. Joel M. Kremer, an associate professor of medicine at Albany Medical College, and his colleagues reported a forty-patient, placebo-controlled, double-blind crossover study.[5] They gave fifteen MaxEPA fish oil capsules daily to twenty patients for fourteen weeks. The patients continued their normal diets with the only difference being the MaxEPA fish oil supplement. At the same time another group of twenty arthritis patients took the same number of placebo capsules.

After the fourteen-week period all forty patients began a four-week washout period in which they took no MaxEPA fish oil or placebo. The groups were then "crossovered"— i.e., for fourteen weeks each group then took the capsules formerly taken by the other group. Another four-week washout period followed. Thirty-three patients completed the clinical trial. Dr. Kremer reports, "Those taking fish oil had only about half the number of tender joints as they had prior to the study, and about half as many as the patients taking the placebo. The benefit vanished during the washout period." The researchers also noted that MaxEPA fish oil slowed the onset of fatigue.

Dr. Kremer also gave an updated report on the study at the 1986 annual meeting of the American Rheumatism Association (ARA) in which he reported that MaxEPA fish oil produced a 60% reduction in LTB4 in humans as well as laboratory animals. The MaxEPA fish oil also increased the production of LTB5 in humans. Dr. Kremer reported, "We saw a significant correlation between the drop in leukotriene B4 and the decrease in the number of tender joints. Those receiving the EPA supplement weren't in as much pain, their joints were less tender and they made it through the day longer before fatigue set in."

Dr. Kremer published his findings in the *Annals of Internal Medicine* in 1987.

Also at the ARA meeting, Dr. Richard I. Sperling, a Harvard associate professor of medicine, reported on a nineteen-patient study. For ten weeks twelve patients were given twenty MaxEPA fish oil capsules daily while seven patients were given a placebo. All patients also received a non-steroidal anti-inflammatory drug during the first six weeks. At the end of the first six weeks the MaxEPA group was found to have significantly fewer tender joints. The benefit disappeared when the drug was withdrawn, but it was significant to note that even without the drug the patients did not deteriorate from their condition at the start of the test, which is what usually happens when the drug is withdrawn.

Dr. Dwight R. Robinson, a rheumatologist at Massachusetts General Hospital, reported that MaxEPA fish oil has the most striking protective effect seen thus far in any animal tests of inflammatory diseases. He found that MaxEPA fish oil was effective in laboratory mice having systemic lupus. The National Institutes of Health conducted a multicentered study of about sixty systemic lupus patients and is preparing to report their results at the time of this writing.

In 1988 an Australian study showed that 18 grams of fish oil a day for three months resulted in fewer sore joints and measurable improvements in grip strength in rheumatoid arthritis patients.[6]

Gamma-linolenic Acid (GLA)

As stated above, the production of the proper prostaglandins requires the proper precursor nutrients. Gamma-linolenic acid (GLA) can be converted by the body into the Family 1 prostaglandins that reduce pain, swelling, and inflammation.

GLA-rich evening primrose oil is effective in controlling rheumatoid arthritis in a substantial number of patients.[7] However, three factors should be noted. First, GLA does not seem to benefit patients receiving more than trivial doses of steroids or indomethacinlike or aspirinlike drugs. This is because they have conflicting action on prostaglandin PGE. However, GLA can be taken and then the drug dosage reduced after one to three months.

Second, the benefits of GLA do not become apparent for one to three months. Some patients experience a transient setback during the first week or two, although they do best in the long run.

Third, there is preliminary evidence that the disease itself may actually be halted in some patients, as opposed to the effects of the action of drugs.

In 1987 a report on evening primrose oil given at the annual meeting of the British Association for Rheumatology and Rehabilitation revealed that 90% of thirty-four arthritis patients who took evening primrose oil felt better within two to four months. More than 80% either stopped taking their anti-inflammatory drugs or cut back on the amount.

Dr. J. Belch and colleagues at the Royal Infirmary at

Glasgow, Scotland have found that GLA and EPA reduce the need for other medication. Rheumatoid arthritis patients were given 540 milligrams of GLA and 240 milligrams of EPA, or 450 milligrams of GLA alone, or a placebo. After a year, patients in the GLA/EPA group or GLA-alone group had verified clinical improvements and had reduced the amount of anti-inflammatory medicine required in comparison to the control group receiving the placebo.[8]

GLA is found in evening primrose oil, borage, and black currants.

Selenium and Vitamin E

As I said before, free radicals as well as prostaglandins cause the pain and inflammation of arthritis. The free radicals may be the first causative step, which is then followed by prostaglandin production as a reaction to the free radicals. The nutritional antioxidants that have been shown to be effective in clinical trials are selenium plus the vitamins A, C, and E. A free-radical scavenger produced in the body, superoxide dismutase, is also beneficial and will be discussed in the next section.

In a May 1980 international meeting of selenium researchers, Norwegian physicians reported the beneficial results of selenium against arthritis: "In rheumatoid arthritis it has been suggested that superoxide radicals and lipoperoxides can be generated in the tissues and accelerate the progression of the disease. Since selenium is a component of the protective enzyme glutathione peroxidase, we determined the blood levels of selenium in a group of twenty-three arthritis patients."[9] The rheumatoid arthritis group did have depressed selenium levels compared to a reference group.

Another physician lecturing at this Second International Symposium on Selenium in Biology and Medicine, Dr. E. Crary of Smyrna, Georgia, had already treated patients having traumatic arthritis with selenium plus the antioxidant vitamins A, C, and E, successfully relieving the pain in their traumatic joints.

In 1982, the British Arthritic Association conducted a three-month clinical trial of a formulation containing selenium plus vitamins A, C, and E. The study included some of the worst cases, and yet 64% reported considerable reduction in pain within the three-month trial period. Many of the volunteers continued the supplement after the formal study period and continued to improve.

Among the patients was Mr. Charles Ware, seventy-four years old, the British Arthritic Association's president, who developed arthritis of the hip after a fall during World War II. He told newspaper reporters, "I thought that I would never get rid of the pain. But now I have full movement of my hip and no pain whatsoever." The British Arthritic Association is now recommending supplements of selenium plus vitamins A, C, and E to all its members.

Following newspaper accounts of this successful clinical trial, the British magazine *Here's Health* distributed this same formulation to a hundred volunteers. The results were so good that they then gave the supplements to 1,000 volunteers. Replies to a follow-up questionnaire were received from 418 of the volunteers. Improvement was noted by 315 (75%).

A Danish study was published in 1985 that confirmed the 1980 Norwegian study. Blood selenium levels were measured in eighty-seven rheumatoid arthritis patients. The researchers, headed by Dr. U. Tarp, found significant differences in selenium levels of patients having three distinct phases of the disease.

The patients having an active, disabling disease of long duration had a very low blood selenium level (65 mcg/l). The group with protracted but mild disease had a moderately low level (74 mcg/l). The group with mild disease of short duration had a slight but statistically significant deficiency (76 mcg/l). The researchers concluded, "A low selenium level may thus be a further factor in the pathogenesis of rheumatoid arthritis."[10] This has been confirmed by four other studies.[11-14]

In Israel a double-blind crossover study in which either 600 milligrams of vitamin E or a placebo was given for ten days to osteoarthritis patients found that more than 50% of the patients had significant relief from pain during the vitamin E period compared to only 4% during the placebo period.

Later Dr. Tarp's group gave 250 micrograms of yeast daily to six volunteers and found no significant improvement above that of the placebo. The researchers concluded that "successful antioxidant therapy for rheumatoid arthritis might require the addition of several free radical scavengers, such as vitamin E and selenium, and the activation of several antioxidant enzyme systems."[15] Yes, that is the point of this section and this book! A synergistic combination is required.

If just one antioxidant is used, the supplementation level must be increased and continued for a longer period of time. The advantage of the synergistic combination is that more enzyme systems are activated and all dosages are within the safety limits. Also, a larger number than six should be considered to measure the effect. The improvement in glutathione peroxidase activity that was detected was ruled insignificant due to the small number of subjects. The same 17% increase would have been significant if the sample group was thirty-six instead of six.

Nutrition Reviews called the results "worthy of note."[16] *Nutrition Reviews* also noted that even after six months of supplementation granulocytes from rheumatoid arthritis patients still had activities below normal. Thus my suggestion for a longer time to first allow the granulocytes to be completely restored to normal and then further time allowed for the action to reduce the inflammation. However, the best approach is to use a synergistic combination of antioxidant nutrients.

Japanese researcher Dr. Masaru Kondo has found that treating arthritis patients with 350 micrograms of selenium and 400 IU of vitamin E daily, plus injections of white blood cells from healthy persons, to be very effective. All seven of his first patients improved dramatically, and by the time he had written his report, five were essentially free from arthritis.[16]

When the white blood cell injections were given without the antioxidant nutrients, only one in thirty patients was essentially free of disease in the same time frame. All patients had severe joint pains for over four years prior to treatment, and their rheumatoid titer factor (RTF) was initially high, averaging 379. The five patients having complete remissions with the antioxidant nutrients had their RTF return to a normal of less than four. The remaining two receiving antioxidant therapy had diminished joint pain and increased joint mobility.

Copper and SOD

Trace amounts of organic-bound copper have helped some individuals. A popular source of such organic copper is superoxide dismutase (SOD). SOD is one of the body's natural free-radical scavengers that reduces pain and inflammation. There is debate as to whether or not SOD itself is absorbed in sufficient quantity to be effective as the inflammation-lowering enzyme SOD—it is when injected—but in any event, the copper may be used to make more of your own SOD.

Dr. Ed Harris of Texas A & M University has shown that low tissue stores of copper cause pain and joint stiffness similar to that of arthritis.[18]

In the 1970s there was a fad of wearing copper bracelets to stop arthritic pain. Although many people experienced reduced pain, they were shamed out of wearing them because this was so unscientific and only folklore. The pain disappearance was explained as being due to the "come and go" nature of the disease.

In one study of patients wearing copper bracelets it was found that people absorbed an average of 13 milligrams of copper during a month. This could bring many people into the recommended daily intake range for copper (1.5 to 3 milligrams). Copper absorbed through the skin gets into circulation very efficiently—more so than most dietary copper. Incidentally, the people absorbing the copper noticed significant improvement in their arthritic conditions as well as a reduction of pain.[19]

Dr. Ray Walker of the University of Newcastle in New South Wales found that thirty-one of forty arthritis patients felt better wearing the copper bracelets. Seventeen patients said there was less pain while they wore the bracelets, and fourteen others said that they were unwilling to carry on for two months without the bracelets.

Dr. Walker was a skeptic and wanted to disprove the suggested link. He had authentic-looking "imitation copper" bracelets made out of aluminum. One group wore copper bracelets and the other group wore lookalike bracelets. Although patients in both groups improved, many more in the copper-bracelet group improved.

Another skeptic, a columnist for a scientific journal, investigated the issue after a scientist reader reported beneficial effects of a copper bracelet on his wife. She had been wearing it but discontinued because it tarnished and turned her skin green. The scientist thought that fatty acids in the skin might be dissolving the oxide on the surface of the bracelet, producing fat-soluble copper "soaps" that could be absorbed through the skin.

The columnist tried the bracelet himself, and his arthritic pains were alleviated. The skin under his bracelet became green. He licked the stain and noted the metallic taste of copper salts. Water alone would not remove the stain. He had to use soap to get it off. He decided that indeed the copper was migrating into his body through his skin.

Isn't it time that someone does a large clinical study, rather than just supposing that it can't work?

Silicon

Clinical studies by Dr. A. Charnot, head of medical research in Morocco, showed a dramatic increase in articular mobility and a marked lessening of pain in the vast majority of those receiving silicon supplementation. He also found that sclerotic areas tended to disappear while decalcified areas tended to recalcify, a frequent finding on X rays.[20]

Dimethylglycine (DMG)

Dr. J. W. Lawson of Clemson University reported that dimethylglycine protected laboratory animals from arthritis induced by an immunological response.[21] Injection of collagen into laboratory rats causes arthritis. The animals produce antibodies to the collagen, which results in an inflammatory process and arthritis. DMG prevents the arthritis from forming.

Nightshades

Some people are allergic or sensitive to foods from the nightshade family. Their sensitivity to these foods is expressed as arthritis. These foods include white potatoes (including potato starch), tomatoes, peppers (except black), and eggplants. These foods contain solanine, which causes delayed inflammation in some persons. If your arthritic condition doesn't respond to anything else, you may wish to abstain from the nightshade foods for about a year.

It is not as easy as it sounds, because these foods can be hidden in prepared foods. Careful label reading is required.

Dr. Norman F. Childers of Rutgers University treated over one thousand arthritis patients successfully with his "no-nightshade diet." A very descriptive book on the relationship between nightshades and arthritis is *Arthritis: Don't Learn to Live with It* by Dr. Carlton Fredericks.[21]

Other foods cause sensitivities manifesting as arthritis. Dr. Richard S. Panush of Saint Barnabas Medical Center in New Jersey found food sensitivities caused 5% of arthritis and aggravated another 30%. The foods were, more often than the nightshades, milk, corn, wheat, beef, fruits, vegetables, and preservatives.

Dr. Panush suggests that the few who do suffer allergic arthritis may wish to fast for three days and then return to a diet free of the suspected foods for a month. In the meantime, monitor pain and joint stiffness and soreness. The delayed allergic reactions produce the inflammation over a period of time, thus a substantial period is needed for the effects to diminish.

Supplements

The nutrients listed in Table 22.1 have been shown to have special value to arthritis patients. You may wish to evaluate several combinations to see if they bring relief to you.

TABLE 22.1
Supplements for Arthritis Sufferers

Nutrient	Daily Amount
Selenium	100–200 mcg
Vitamin E	400–800 IU
Fish oil	500–8,000 mg
Evening primrose oil (GLA)	3,000–4,000 mg
Vitamin C	500–3,000 mg
Copper	1–2 mg
Zinc	15–25 mg
Magnesium	400–600 mg
Calcium	250–500 mg
Silicon	5–25 mg
Dimethylglycine (DMG)	100–250 mg
Pycnogenol	50–150 mg

23

Diabetes

The incidence of diabetes has risen over 600% in little more than one generation. An estimated one out of every twenty Americans will become diabetic. Diabetes is the third leading cause of death in the U.S., accounting for 300,000 to 350,000 deaths each year. Diabetes also contributes to the development of other deadly diseases. It is estimated that one half of those with coronary artery disease and three quarters of stroke victims developed their circulatory problems prematurely as a result of diabetes.

Diabetes is a disorder in which the body cannot convert foods properly into energy. Actually diabetes may be a group of diseases having various causes but all resulting in a decrease in the body's ability to handle blood sugar normally. The word "diabetes" is based on a Greek word meaning "to pass through." Diabetes mellitus is the most common form of diabetes. "Mellitus" is derived from a Greek word that means "honey-sweet." Diabetes mellitus denotes the disease first described in 1500 B.C. of persons with honey-sweet-tasting urine. We can ignore the details, but sixth-century physicians in India thought that the honey-sweet-tasting urine was produced by sugar passing through the body unchanged. In the seventeenth century an English scientist, Thomas Willis, was credited with being the first to advise diabetics not to eat sweets.

In the eighteenth century it was shown that diabetics had excess sugar in both their urine and their blood. By 1901 it was shown that the problem was often due to an impairment in the islandlike cluster of cells in the pancreas called the islets of Langerhans. By the 1920s it was found that most cases of diabetes could be controlled by insulin, a substance secreted by the islets.

When a person eats sugars and starches the body changes them rapidly into a sugar called glucose, which is circulated in the blood for immediate use or is converted into glycogen and stored in muscles and the liver for later use as a quick source of energy.

In diabetes, the mechanism that controls the amount of glucose in the blood breaks down. The blood glucose level then increases to a dangerously high level, causing symptoms and damage to the body. This buildup occurs either because the body does not have enough insulin or because the insulin is not fully effective on the body tissues.

After a meal, a diabetic's blood glucose (blood sugar) level can exceed 300 milligrams per 100 milliliters of blood. The normal range is 60 to 100 milligrams of glucose per 100 milliliters of blood. The large amount of glucose circulating in the bloodstream can damage sensitive kidney tubes, making them porous to sugars and proteins that then spill into the urine. This process causes the kidneys to excrete a large amount of urine, and thus the body loses a lot of water. Naturally, then, common symptoms of diabetes are abnormal thirst and frequent urination.

There are two main types of diabetes. Type 1, or "insulin-dependent" diabetes, is the more severe form of the disease. Although this type of diabetes can appear at any age, it generally starts during childhood or adolescence. Usually lifelong treatment via insulin injections is required, along with diet control and exercise.

Before the introduction of insulin as a therapeutic agent most severe Type 1 diabetics would die in diabetic coma—an episode of acute insulin insufficiency leading to massive elevations of blood sugar, loss of blood volume (circulatory hypovolemia), shock (secondary to the resulting osmotic diuresis), acidosis (due to the buildup of ketone bodies), coma, and death.

Diabetic coma is far less common now as a cause of death since it can be managed by sufficiently prompt insulin administration. *However, many other complications of long-standing diabetes are not readily prevented by insulin therapy.* Standard insulin treatments cannot prevent intermittent elevations of blood sugar that cause damage to filtering mechanisms of the kidney called glomeruli (with resultant high blood pressure), to the retinal arteries and the eye lens (sometimes resulting in blindness), and to the peripheral nervous system (causing pain, tingling, anesthesia, and motor defects).

This damage occurs in tissues whose glucose (sugar) content tends to reflect that of the blood, and it is thought to result from osmotic damage or accumulation of the glucose metabolite sorbitol, or even from excess blood sugar attachment to red blood cells, the lining of blood vessels, or the insulating material (myelin) around nerve cells.

Rapid increases in blood sugar resulting from eating quickly assimilated refined carbohydrates will lead to a corresponding high secretion of insulin and glucose tolerance factor (GTF). Much of this secreted GTF will be lost into the urine. Thus, refined diets increase the need for chromium, which is needed to make GTF.

It is also believed that peaks of blood sugar and insulin caused by rapid intestinal absorption may result in a reflex end-organ insensitivity to insulin.

When the diet consists of slowly absorbed, complex, fiber-rich and chromium-GTF-rich carbohydrates, and when glucose tolerance is excellent, there is little need for fat as a metabolic fuel. The body's homeostatic recognition of this fact results in low blood cholesterol and triglyceride levels and a decreased incidence of heart disease.

Non-Insulin-dependent

The common form of diabetes that strikes mostly adults is Type II, or non–insulin-dependent diabetes. Previously known as adult-onset diabetes, this form of the disease accounts for over 85% of all diabetes cases. Most people with this type of diabetes do not need insulin injections. They can usually keep their blood sugar level near normal by such "prudent" measures as controlling their weight, exercising, and following a diet low in simple carbohydrates (sugars). Obesity and lack of exercise, which for unknown reasons produce a further impairment of glucose tolerance, are now more common in our modern society.

Recent research has shown that some increase in blood sugar levels may occur normally with age. The National Institute on Aging has proposed that the diagnostic standards for detecting diabetes be changed so that an older person's performance on the blood glucose test may be judged against the performance of other older people and not against that of younger individuals. By interpreting the blood glucose test in this way, fewer persons will be incorrectly diagnosed as being diabetic.

A panel of experts brought together by the National Institutes of Health recently recommended such an adjustment in diagnostic standards. This recommendation, which applies to all age groups, has been widely accepted by physicians specializing in the treatment of diabetes.

If an adult has abnormally high levels of blood sugar even when compared in this improved way, the first step is to measure the amount of insulin that is available in the blood. If the pancreas is producing adequate insulin, then something must be interfering with the body's ability to use that insulin. Poor insulin utilization can be caused by such factors as: the insulin not attaching itself to its receptors on cell surfaces; insufficient numbers of insulin receptors on cell surfaces; blocked insulin receptors; destroyed insulin receptors due to disease, physical damage, or repeated insulin floodings; poor transport of the chemical messengers inside the cells that are released when insulin attaches itself to its receptors; or incorrect timing of the release of insulin.

One line of research indicates that free radicals can destroy the insulin-producing beta cells of the pancreas. Antioxidant nutrients can reduce this damage and thus help prevent diabetes.[1]

Chromium

The common link between heart disease and diabetes is a chromium deficiency. The glucose tolerance factor (GTF) contains chromium. GTF potentiates the action of endogenously produced insulin secreted in response to physiological need. For this reason, the progression of end-organ insensitivity, a common flaw with standard insulin therapy, may be less likely to develop with GTF supplementation.

As early as 1966 Dr. Walter Mertz of the USDA Human Research Center in Beltsville, Maryland reported that chromium helped diabetics. Since then several clinical trials have adequately confirmed the role of chromium in improving glucose tolerance in diabetics.

Dr. Esther Offenbacher found that the GTF in nine grams of brewer's yeast taken daily for two months improved glucose tolerance while decreasing insulin need in elderly patients.[2] (Chromium-poor torula yeast was also tested and found not to produce similar improvement.)

Dr. Offenbacher noted that "an improvement in insulin sensitivity also occurred with brewer's yeast supplementation. This supports the thesis that elderly people may have a low level of chromium and that an effective source for chromium repletion, such as brewer's yeast, may improve their carbohydrate tolerance and blood fats."

Elderly people are of special interest because they are more prone to diabetes (and chromium depletion). It has been estimated that 40% to 60% of eighty-year-olds have diabetes.

Earlier studies by Dr. Richard Doisy revealed that 150 micrograms of inorganic chromium improved glucose tolerance in 40% of elderly patients with glucose intolerance.[3] These findings confirmed still earlier observations by Dr. C. M. McCay.[4]

As Dr. Doisy pointed out: "Possibly some individuals (i.e. insulin-requiring diabetics) completely lose their ability to convert chromium to GTF. The daily dietary intake of chromium and GTF is quite variable depending on the nature of the diet selected. If it is true, as suggested (by the evidence), that the insulin-requiring diabetic is unable to convert chromium to GTF, then the insulin-requiring diabetic would be dependent solely on the exogenous GTF in the diet. This could explain the so-called "brittle diabetics." If GTF intake is high one day, the insulin requirement is reduced. Conversely, if GTF intake is low, the insulin requirement is increased. By feeding brewer's yeast daily, the daily GTF intake is more constant and thus insulin dosage may remain more constant. It may be worthy of mention that a few of the insulin-requiring diabetics have reported a greater stability of blood sugar with less tendency to spill sugar over into the urine and a reduced incidence of hypoglycemic reactions while on the brewer's yeast supplement."

In working with a strain of laboratory mice that are genetically diabetic I found that chromium-GTF supplements halted the pathology of the diabetes and greatly increased their life spans.

It appears that in insulin-dependent diabetics a greater percentage of their dietary chromium is excreted than in non-diabetics.[5] A new chromium supplement, chromium picolinate, has been shown to be very effective in Type 2 diabetics, in which diminished tissue responsiveness to insulin is the primary defect. Dr. Gary Evans of Bemidji State University, in collaboration with Drs. Richard Press and J. Geller, found that Type 2 diabetics given 200 micrograms of chromium daily in the form of 1.6 milligrams of chromium picolinate reduced fasting blood sugar 18% and glycosylated hemoglobin by 10%.[6]

Vitamin E

The alteration in blood platelets that was discussed in Chapter 18 contributes to the circulatory problems and heart disease common to diabetics. Diabetics have an increased tendency for altered blood platelets and clotting. Vitamin E inhibits platelet aggregation and sticky blood as explained in Chapter 18.

Dr. Claude Colette and colleagues at the Hospital Lapeyromie in France demonstrated that vitamin E does indeed help Type 1 (insulin-dependent) diabetics. One gram

(1,000 milligrams) of vitamin E daily produced a small but significant reduction in platelet aggregation in the diabetics.[7]

Furthermore, other researchers have shown that vitamin E improves other factors in diabetics that are related to blood clotting and circulation. Diabetics produce more thromboxane A-2, which increases clotting. Dr. C. Gisinger and colleagues found that 400 IU of vitamin E daily reduced blood platelet aggregation and thromboxane A-2 production.[8]

Studies on diabetics at the University of Kentucky by Dr. I. Chen and R. Thacker indicated that vitamin C and vitamin E play important and independent roles to reduce heart disease risk.[9]

Pyridoxine Alpha-ketoglutarate (PAK)

Wow! That's a mouthful. Three cheers for the three-letter designation system we lazy chemists came up with. This is the first time that I have discussed PAK in detail in this book. PAK is under active research for its role in energy output and insulin potentiation. Italian researchers have found that PAK's ability to reduce lactic acid buildup, which is the result of muscles working, is an aid to diabetics and athletes alike.[10]

When blood sugar is metabolized to produce energy, one of the waste products is lactic acid. When lactic acid accumulates in the muscle cells, the muscles tire because the energy-producing reactions are slowed by the lactic acid buildup. The lactic acid can even make the muscles "burn" if they are forced to continue working, as is the case for many weight lifters and bodybuilders who exercise until the muscles "burn." Diabetics produce lactic acid at the same rate as non-diabetics, but diabetics don't remove lactic acid from the muscle as quickly.

Disposal of lactic acid is not so much a "transport" problem as a "degradation" problem. The best way to solve a lactic acid buildup is to take care of it right in the cells producing it. Diabetics differ from non-diabetics in how they break up the lactic acid molecule. As the cells break down the lactic acid molecules into smaller chemical units of carbon compounds, some degradation products are used in the cell to make carbon dioxide, and some are used to make blood sugar, which recycles to produce more energy. Type 1 diabetics tend to recycle a greater percentage of the breakdown products back into blood sugar, but at a slower rate.[11] PAK promotes this conversion more quickly, thus normalizing the ability of diabetics to utilize their muscles for work or exercise.[12]

An important aspect is that PAK improves blood sugar and the glucose tolerance test in both Type 1 and Type 2 diabetics.[13] The researchers concluded that PAK "potentiated the effects of insulin . . . and enhanced glucose metabolism and pyruvate oxidation."

Quercetin

Quercetin improves the functioning of the islet cells of the pancreas, thereby improving the release of insulin.[14] Quercetin has been shown to prevent some of the major complications of diabetes, including cataracts, diabetic retinopathy (blindness), neuropathy (nerve damage), and nephropathy (kidney damage).[15,16]

Fish Oil

One would expect that fish oils would be beneficial to diabetics because they reduce heart and artery diseases that are associated with diabetes. However, the clinical evidence is so mixed that a conclusion cannot be made at this time. The subject must be discussed, pro and con, to alert diabetics who may be trying to protect themselves against the side effects of diabetes that fish oils may do more harm than good—or vice versa.

Pro

Research has shown that fish oil helps non-insulin diabetics (type 2) utilize their own insulin. Type 2 diabetics frequently develop the disease as a result of obesity, and their insulin loses some of its effect in controlling blood sugar.

Dutch researchers have found that 30 grams of MaxEPA daily improves Type 2 diabetics' blood sugar control.[17]

Dr. Margaret J. Albrink, professor of medicine at West Virginia University in Morgantown, examined whether the beneficial cardiovascular effects of fish oils applied to diabetics as well.[18] She found that very large amounts of fish oil (45 milliliters, which contains nearly 18 grams of omega-3 fatty acids) produced dramatic reductions of blood triglycerides and cholesterol and returned platelet aggregation to normal without changing the bleeding time.

Fish oil enhances insulin sensitivity and thus should be protective against heart disease and diabetes, according to research at Loyola University of New Orleans by Dr. E. I. Beard and colleagues.[19]

Con

However, a ten-week study at the Royal Perth Hospital in Western Australia indicates that it is possible, but not certain, that Type 1 diabetics may have an altered metabolic response to EPA. A mixture of beneficial and detrimental lipoprotein changes were observed by the group headed by Dr. T. A. Mori.

The Type 1 diabetics showed significant decreases in blood triglyceride levels, but also significant increases in blood cholesterol, LDL, and HDL levels. Diabetics should monitor their blood cholesterol, LDL, and HDL if they take fish oil.

The Australian researchers found that 15 grams of fish oil daily was not associated with any change in nonfasting blood sugar, glycosylated hemoglobin, or insulin requirements in diabetics.[20]

A study conducted by Dr. John Esnick of the University School of Medicine on six Type 2 diabetics who took eight grams of fish oil daily for eight weeks found that their blood sugar level increased an average of 20%, while the insulin secreted was less.[21]

Another study of six diabetics by Dr. Harry Glauber of the University of California at San Diego found essentially the same results.[22]

Until we know more, diabetics should take fish oil supplements only under the care of a physician who monitors blood chemistry closely.

Zinc

Zinc is a component of insulin. Diabetics should facilitate their production of insulin by being sure they are not deficient in zinc. Even a 1% reduction in insulin production due to a severe zinc deficiency could be harmful.

A study at Wayne State University led by zinc researcher Ananda Prasad found that diabetics were lower in zinc than healthy persons. The researchers suggested that several diabetic complications may be related to low zinc status, including slow healing of ulcers, neurosensory changes, low testosterone levels, and impaired immune function.[23]

Supplements

Diabetics may wish to improve their total diet and consider the supplements listed in Table 23.1.

Insulin-dependent diabetics making dietary changes are very likely to change their insulin needs. If you are a Type 1, you should be sure to monitor blood sugar levels closely to prevent insulin shock or diabetic coma. As diabetics know so well, insulin shock results from having too much insulin circulating in the blood because you haven't eaten as many calories as needed or your body has become more efficient in using insulin. Diabetic coma results when the blood sugar level gets too high because of too many calories or not enough insulin.

TABLE 23.1
Supplements for Diabetics

Nutrient	Daily Amount
Vitamin E	400–800 IU
Vitamin C	500–2,000 mg
Chromium (GTF or picolinate)	150–300 mcg
Quercetin	100–300 mg
Zinc	15–25 mg
Pyridoxine-alpha-ketoglutarate (PAK)	(3 × 600) 1,800 mg

24

PMS and Cystic Mastitis

Women have to put up with so much discomfort and special risks, yet on the average, women outlive men by seven or eight years.

"Big, tough" men sometimes think that those of the "weaker gender" tend to be hypochondriacs. The thought would never again cross their minds if they had premenstrual syndrome, gave birth, or went through menopause. The problem used to be called premenstrual tension but is now usually called premenstrual syndrome (PMS).

Personally, I liked the description "premenstrual tension" better because it described the cause—increased tension due to water retention—and the effect—increased emotional tension. The increased water retention would surely cause physical discomfort, but the brain tissue swelling in the confines of the skull also causes emotional discomfort. Men often refer to the resulting personality change as "the old changed-into-a-witch-overnight syndrome." Sometimes they misspell "witch" with a "b."

One of the first special discomforts experienced by women are those irritating annoyances occurring about a week or two (luteal phase) before their menstrual period—the bloating, cramps, tender breasts, headaches, backache, abdominal discomfort, hot flushes, abnormal thirst, fatigue, dizziness, and mood swings of irritability, depression, anger, hostility, and anxiety. Other less common symptoms include a craving for sweets, appetite and sex drive changes, and even flare-ups in acne, herpes, asthma, and other disorders. These symptoms affect about half of menstruating women, with about 5% to 10% severely affected.

There are four recognized symptom categories of PMS, each having its own symptoms. A woman may suffer from any combination of the symptom categories. The categories were developed by Dr. Guy E. Abraham and are classified PMS-A (anxiety), PMS-H (hyperhydration [water retention]), PMS-C (cravings), and PMS-D (depression). Approximately 75% to 80% of women suffer the symptoms of PMS-A, 60% to 70% suffer with PMS-H, 35% to 40% suffer with PMS-C symptoms, and 30% to 35% have PMS-D symptoms. Table 24.1 lists the categories and their symptoms. A typical woman may have two or three of the symptom categories.

The purpose of classifying the symptoms into categories is to facilitate treatment of the symptoms. The "alternative" strategy is to treat the cause, not the symptoms. This chapter lists the nutrients that will balance the hormones and prostaglandins that cause the symptoms. If you are properly nourished, you won't cycle out of balance.

TABLE 24.1
PMS Categories and Their Symptoms

PMS-A Anxiety, nervous tension, irritability, mood swings

PMS-H Water retention (abdominal bloating and tenderness), breast tenderness, weight gain, swelling of feet and hands

PMS-C Cravings (sweets, chocolates), increased appetite, headaches, fainting, heart palpitations

PMS-D Depression, confusion, fatigue, crying, forgetfulness, insomnia

---

The standard therapies that treat the symptoms rather than the cause include painkillers, diuretics, hormones, and tranquilizers. However, this may be a case where the cure is worse than the disease due to addiction and nutritional depletion.

The number of women experiencing PMS is increasing, probably as a result of suboptimal nutrition and/or contraceptive pill usage. Modern low-calorie diets required to maintain one's figure in these sedentary times are also low in vitamin B-6, magnesium, calcium, and other vital nutrients. "The Pill" depletes one's levels of vitamin B-6, folic acid, and certain other nutrients. The resultant nutritional deficiencies lead to an imbalance between the hormones progesterone and estrogen blood levels, which in turn produce atypical release of brain compounds such as beta-endorphins and other peptides.

Caffeine and caffeinelike compounds (theophylline in tea and theobromine in chocolate) have been implicated in PMS by several studies. I have had many reports from women who find rapid improvement when they eliminate caffeine.

A study at Oregon State University by Dr. Annette MacKay Rossignol examined 188 tea drinkers, of which 52% experienced marked PMS. She found that women who drank four to eight cups of tea daily had five times the PMS symptoms of those who drank less. Caffeine may not exacerbate the PMS symptoms in all women, but it surely seems to have an effect on some.

More will be said about caffeine in the section on cystic mastitis later in this chapter.

Aerobic exercise is important. Not just during the period of symptoms, but regular exercise. Brisk walking for thirty minutes every other day will do much for preventing or at least reducing the severity of PMS symptoms.

A study by Dr. R. London and colleagues at the Homewood Hospital Center in Maryland of sixty PMS sufferers showed that women taking a multiple-vitamin, multiple-mineral supplement have fewer PMS symptoms. The women were divided into three groups. One group received a placebo, a second group received multiple-vitamin, multiple-mineral supplements, and a third group half vitamins and minerals and half placebo.

The placebo group had no significant reduction in symptoms. The vitamin-mineral group did have significant reductions in irritability, tension, depression, motor coordination, and menstrual symptoms.

A similar study was conducted in England by the Pre-Menstrual Tension Advisory Service in Hove. The study was reported in 1987 by Dr. A. Stewart.[1] The four-month study involved a placebo group, a low-dose multivitamin, multi-mineral supplement, and a high-dose multivitamin, multi-mineral.

The low-dosage "multi" did only slightly better than the placebo in reducing PMS symptoms. The high-dosage "multi" did considerably better than the placebo, with 71% of the women reporting improvement. Dr. Stewart concluded, "nutritional deficiencies could influence symptomatology, and that correction of these deficiencies is a logical first step in the management of PMS."

Let's look at how specific nutrients help correct the imbalances that cause the various PMS symptoms.

Magnesium

PMS patients have been found to have significantly low levels of magnesium in their red blood cells in comparison to women not suffering from PMS. A study at the Sussex County Hospital and the Well Woman Clinic in East Sussex, England examined the magnesium levels of the plasma and red blood cells of 105 women suffering from PMS. The PMS patients had lower plasma and red blood cell magnesium levels, with approximately half of the PMS patients having red blood cell magnesium levels below the lower limit of the normal range.[2]

In the U.S. Dr. Guy Abraham has found that magnesium helps all types of PMS patients.[3]

Vitamin E

Vitamin E is also helpful because it inhibits the formation of the undesirable leukotrienes. Dr. Robert London of the Sinai Hospital in Baltimore and Johns Hopkins University School of Medicine found that 300 IU of vitamin E significantly improved all PMS categories except PMS-H.[4]

Four years later Dr. London and his colleagues conducted another clinical trial to confirm the results of the first. Women given 400 IU of vitamin E daily for three months reported an average 33% reduction in physical symptoms, 38% reduction in anxiety, and a 27% improvement in depression. The women also reported less fatigue, fewer headaches, and a decrease in cravings for sweets.[5]

The study was a placebo-controlled study in which twenty-two women received the vitamin E and nineteen women received a placebo. Five women dropped out of the study because they were not noticing benefits. Four of the five women were taking the placebo, not the vitamin E.

The researchers concluded that vitamin E supplementation is a rational approach to the management of PMS. "The results of the present investigation are consistent with our previous observations that alpha-tocopherol (vitamin E) supplementation reduces symptoms of PMS, with no demonstrable side effects."

At a 1986 seminar on vitamin E Dr. Helmuth Vorherr of the University of New Mexico reported that vitamin E was producing benefits within four months in women given 800 IU of natural vitamin E daily.[6]

Notice that in the above two studies vitamin E was given for three and four months before the evaluations. Remember, correcting nutritional imbalances takes a while. It is not the same as taking an aspirin for a headache. My experience with the vitamin E study that I conducted in 1976 and other observations since is that the improvement continues with time. I suggest that if the evaluation were given after six months, the improvement would be even greater. To get a feeling for the time effect with vitamin E, review my vitamin E study findings in Chapter 18 on heart disease and Chapter 9 on menopause.

Vitamin B-6

Vitamin B-6 has brought relief to women suffering from PMS since the 1940s, but physicians have only recognized this as fact since a series of clinical trials confirmed it using the manner of testing that they trust. In 1980 a six-month study was published in *Infertility* that showed that 500 milligrams of vitamin B-6 daily relieved PMS in twenty-one of the twenty-five women in the placebo-controlled clinical trial.

In 1987 a study involving fifty-five PMS sufferers found that 150 milligrams of vitamin B-6 reduced PMS symptoms such as dizziness, nausea, and behavioral changes such as poor performance or withdrawal from social activities.[7]

Dr. M. Brush and colleagues at the St. Thomas Hospital and Medical School in London reported on their seven-year study of 630 PMS patients.[8,9] The PMS patients were treated with 40 to 200 milligrams of vitamin B-6 daily. Forty percent of the women receiving from 100 to 150 milligrams of vitamin B-6 daily experienced significant reductions in symptoms. However, 60% of those receiving from 160 to 200 milligrams of vitamin B-6 daily showed significant improvements. Many of the patients receiving lower amounts of vitamin B-6 also showed partial improvement. No side effects were reported, and no peripheral neuropathy was detected.

Symptoms that were significantly reduced included depression, irritability, anxiety, tension, fluid retention, headache, breast tenderness, cravings, lethargy, and others.

Almost identical findings were reported by Dr. M. Williams and colleagues in a study of 600 women involving eighty-five general practitioners in England.[10] The dosages and times were the same, and the results were the same. Again, no side effects were observed.

We should not be surprised at the effectiveness of vitamin B-6 now that we better understand the interrelationships between vitamin B-6, prostaglandins, and the symptoms of PMS. Vitamin B-6 is needed for the conversion of cis-linoleic acid to gamma-linolenic acid (GLA) and thence to prostaglandin E-1. Prostaglandin E-1 is the good prostaglandin that has a diuretic action, reduces pain, and reduces inflammation. Prostaglandin E-1 deficiency also increases sensitivity to the hormone prolactin.

Don't try to get even more relief by taking larger and larger quantities of vitamin B-6. There is evidence that very large amounts of vitamin B-6 can cause tingling sensations in the arms in some women. While 500 milligrams daily may be without side effects in most women, it can cause side effects in some. A few are sensitive even at 200 milligrams per day. It is reasonable to limit vitamin B-6 intake to no more than 200 milligrams per day unless advised otherwise by your physician. If side effects occur, check with your physician.

Gamma-linolenic Acid (GLA)

PMS patients have been shown to have a slight defect in their ability to convert cis-linoleic acid into gamma-linolenic acid (GLA). Taking GLA directly in a food source such as evening primrose oil bypasses the dependence of prostaglandin production on vitamin B-6.

Dr. David Horrobin of the Efamol Research Institute in Kentville, Nova Scotia reported six successful clinical trials of evening primrose oil in PMS patients.[11]

One study of sixty-eight PMS patients was supervised by Dr. M. G. Brush of the Department of Gynecology at St. Thomas's Hospital Medical School in London. This is the largest university PMS clinic in Britain. All of the women in the study had failed to respond to at least one conventional therapy for PMS, and most of the patients had failed to respond to two conventional treatment programs. Of these very difficult patients, 61% experienced total remission of all symptoms, while an additional 23% had partial relief.

In another study headed by Dr. Brush, blood samples were analyzed from forty-two patients attending a premenstrual syndrome clinic. The blood samples were found to be deficient in GLA and all metabolites of GLA, whereas linoleic acid levels were significantly elevated.[12]

Two additional double-blind, placebo-controlled studies at the University Hospital of Wales, Cardiff, and University of Dundee, Scotland showed similar results. These two studies were primarily concerned with PMS and breast irregularities such as tenderness or cystic nodules, and they will be discussed later in this chapter under cystic mastitis.

A double-blind, placebo-controlled crossover study at the Department of Obstetrics, Helsinki University, Finland also confirmed the effectiveness of evening primrose oil (GLA) against PMS.

A study by British physicians Drs. A. Davies and R. Morse of 196 PMS patients found that irritability was relieved in 77%, depression in 74%, breast pain and tenderness in 76%, headache in 71%, and ankle swelling in 63%.

Dr. Horrobin estimates, based on his twelve years experience with GLA and other nutrients against PMS, that the combined nutritional approach will relieve 95% of PMS patients.

Calcium

A study at the New York Medical College found that calcium supplements reduced PMS symptoms. After three months 72% of the women taking calcium supplements reported having much less pain, water retention, and mood swings, as compared to only 15% of the women receiving the placebo. This study will be expanded, and several dosage levels of calcium will be used.

Supplements to Relieve PMS

You may wish to consider adding the nutrients listed in Table 24.2 to your daily diet (not just during the period of PMS symptoms) to prevent the symptoms of premenstrual syndrome.

CYSTIC MASTITIS

Painful lumps in the breast have caused needless fear in women. The condition is known by several names: cystic

TABLE 24.2
Supplements for PMS

Nutrient	Daily Amount
Evening primrose oil (GLA)	4–8 capsules
Vitamin B-6	50–200 mg
Vitamin C	250–500 mg
Vitamin E	100–400 IU
Niacin	25–100 mg
Pantothenic acid	100–250 mg
Bioflavonoids	50–500 mg
Magnesium	200–400 mg
Calcium	100–250 mg
Zinc	15–25 mg
L-tyrosine	100–250 mg
Choline	25–75 mg
Inositol	25–75 mg

mastitis, fibrocystic breast disease, mammary dysplasia, benign breast disease, and proliferate breast disease. The condition affects 60% of women at one time or another. No matter what you call it, it can be relieved. There's more good news—it's not a risk factor for breast cancer.

A word of caution before you waste time trying to relieve cystic mastitis: Make sure that this is what you have! If you have any lump, check with your doctor right away. Most lumps are harmless, but your life is too important to play the odds. Be sure! If your doctor finds that you are prone to cystic mastitis, then the two of you can work out a system of testing for benign lumps and breast cancer. By the way, when was your last mammogram?

A study by Drs. William Dupont and David Page of Vanderbilt University School of Medicine found that most women (70%) with cystic mastitis are not at increased risk for breast cancer.[13] The 30% of women who also have a family history of breast cancer or who have unusual lesions may be at increased risk.

One problem with cystic mastitis, in addition to the pain, is that the lumps make detection of other lumps more difficult. Hence, mammograms are a necessity.

Why do I mention the good news about breast cancer risk? Back in 1980 *Newsweek* and major newspapers were touting the benefit of removing breasts as a prophylactic against breast cancer. One surgeon had performed over one hundred such operations. Another claimed that he had saved a life by removing the breasts of a fourteen-year-old girl. Thank goodness that this couldn't become a ritual at birth like circumcision. (I must admit that if all breasts were removed, the incidence of breast cancer would be decreased.)

Diet has its effect on the formation of the painful lumps. Caffeine and other members of the methylxanthine family (theophylline in tea and theobromine in chocolate) are strongly linked to cystic mastitis. These compounds are all called caffeine by most people, but they are different. Eliminating coffee, tea, non-decaffeinated colas, and cocoa will eliminate or greatly reduce cystic mastitis in a large percentage of women.

There was one study that indicated that caffeine was not linked to cystic mastitis.[14] However, this study was flawed in that it considered a reduction in "caffeine" by 50% as having complied with the diet. A greater reduction—essentially the elimination—of "caffeine" is required if this is the only approach used.

However, if vitamin E supplementation is also used, the caffeine need not be entirely eliminated. In fact, vitamin E produces good results even when caffeine is not reduced.

Vitamin E

Dr. Robert London, mentioned earlier in this chapter, found that on 600 IU of vitamin E daily 85% of patients in a double-blind placebo-controlled study showed dramatic remission of lumps, and the remaining 15% showed clear improvement. *This is 100% of patients markedly improved with vitamin E.*[15]

Earlier this medical research group described the management of cystic mastitis with 1,000 to 1,500 IU of vitamin E.[16]

Dr. London's group has also found that synthetic vitamin E (d,1-alpha-tocopherol) was ineffective. The only vitamin E that produced the results was natural vitamin E (d-alpha-tocopherol).

In a study with twenty-nine cystic mastitis patients Dr. A. Abrams of the Boston University School of Medicine found that vitamin E supplementation brought about complete relief or significant improvement in all.[17]

Iodine

Dr. Bernard Eskin of the Medical College of Pennsylvania determined that iodine caseinate was very effective against cystic mastitis. Dr. Eskin's thesis is that when iodine is deficient in the diet, estrogen hastens the development of cystic mastitis and breast cancer.

High breast cancer mortality rates are found in the states bordering the Great Lakes. All of the significantly high breast cancer–rate counties are within the iodine-deficient goiter belt or the New-Jersey-to-Massachusetts strip.

The importance of iodine may be related to the thyroid hormone thyroxine, which helps govern the rate of metabolism. The rate of metabolism influences the degradation of estrogen to estriol.

In any event, Dr. Eskin found that 90% of 588 cystic mastitis patients had good-to-excellent results with iodine caseinate. Complete pain relief was reported by 43% of the women.

A follow-up study using diatomic iodine (I_2) found that 95% of 1,300 cystic mastitis patients dramatically improved. Diatomic iodine is *not* the antiseptic tincture of iodine, which is poisonous. Dr. William Ghent of Queen's University in Ontario collaborated with Dr. Eskin in this study. After taking the diatomic iodine for a year 95% had complete relief from pain and lumps. Dr. Ghent has found that long-standing cystic mastitis requires about three years for complete remission.

The researchers also found that if the women stopped taking the diatomic iodine, the lumps would return in as little as a week in some women and within nine months in 90% of the women.

Iodized salt contains iodine, but salt can increase PMS in some women and, as discussed in Chapter 21, can elevate blood pressure in some women. Kelp is an excellent source of iodine that is available as a supplement.

Supplements for Cystic Mastitis

The supplements listed in Table 24.3 should be considered for relief from cystic mastitis.

TABLE 24.3
Supplements for Cystic Mastitis

Nutrient	Daily Amount
Vitamin E	600–800 IU
Kelp (iodine)	as labeled
Choline	25–75 mg
Inositol	25–75 mg

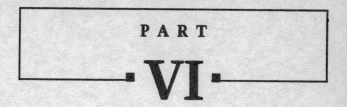

PART

VI

Completing the Supernutrition Story

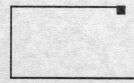
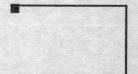

25

Vitamin C and the Common Cold

———————————————◼———————————————

Last, and most certainly least, of the diseases to be discussed in this book is the common cold. A cold or flu is usually not deadly and is only a temporary discomfort, unless the victim is extremely young or elderly. There are two reasons why I am including a short discussion here. First of all, it can cause economic loss or personal disappointment. Secondly, the topic was included in *Supernutrition: Megavitamin Therapy* and has been in and out of the news for years. You deserve an update on the latest facts.

The keys to preventing a cold or flu are as follows:

1. Be well-nourished.
2. Do not get overtired.
3. Do not get depressed.
4. Don't become immersed in an infected group.
5. Wash your hands much more frequently during cold and flu season.

You can be assured that if you are not eating right, are tired and depressed, and walk into a germ-filled room, you will catch a cold or flu. Why? Because your immune system will be depressed. Germs don't cause diseases. The failure of your immune system to destroy germs causes disease. If your immune system is functioning optimally, you won't catch a cold unless you drown yourself in germs.

Statistics say that the average person may have three or four colds a year. I get a cold once every three or four years. I get a flu every six or seven years. When I do feel a cold coming on I stop it in its tracks by taking two grams of vitamin C immediately and one gram every hour until I go to bed. That's the end of it.

Some may say that this is not a nutritional use of vitamin C. Dr. Linus Pauling has pointed out in his writings that 10,000 mg of vitamin C per day is the proper nutritional amount, and that human beings who take less than that are just undernourished. But as a screwdriver can be used to pry open a paint can lid as well as turn a screw, vitamin C can be used for more than one purpose in the body. The body recognizes the vitamin C molecule, not its title.

Being well-nourished with vitamin C reduces the incidence of colds in normal life, and massive amounts of vitamin C reduce the symptoms of colds.

Sure, studies have shown that vitamin C has no effect on colds, but those studies were flawed. Better-designed studies show that vitamin C has a significant effect.

If a study intended to examine conventional resistance to colds induces the germs by squirting enormous amounts of germs up the subject's nose, expect the immune system to be overwhelmed. But this is not how we catch cold in real life.

Also, if the immune system needs a quick stimulation, don't expect a trace of vitamin C once a day to do the job, and don't expect the effect to occur two minutes after the first supplement is taken.

I will only discuss the latest study available at this printing. This is not a balanced discussion, but there is little sense in discussing studies that are not adequately designed.

Dr. Linus Pauling, in his book *How to Live Longer and Feel Better*,[1] cites sixteen well-designed studies indicating that vitamin C decreases the degree of suffering by an average of 34%—and in some people by as much as 68%.

Dr. Elliot Dick and colleagues at the University of Wisconsin conducted a well-designed, double-blind, placebo-controlled study with sixteen healthy volunteers.[2] Half of them received 2,000 milligrams of vitamin C daily split into four portions of 500 milligrams each. The remaining half received a placebo on an identical schedule.

The volunteers were given three weeks to build up the stimulatory effect in their system, and their blood levels of vitamin C were monitored as a check on assimilation and compliance. Then the sixteen volunteers were housed for a week together with eight others having bad colds.

Seven of the eight volunteers on the placebo came down with colds, and six of the eight on vitamin C developed colds. That is not that great of a change, but look at the great difference in severity.

The colds were much milder in the vitamin C group. The vitamin C group had colds that lasted for an average of only seven days, whereas the placebo group had colds averaging twelve days. Plus, the cold symptoms in the vitamin C group were much milder. The number of coughs was cut to a third, sneezes were cut in half, and the number of "nose blows" was cut by a third.

Another study has uncovered part of the mechanism in which vitamin C exerts its protective effect.[3]

A milder cold is harder to spread. So if your friend has a cold, it will help protect you if you lessen the severity of your friend's cold with vitamin C. Spread the word and protect yourself.

26

Safety of Supplements

The safety of food supplements is well established. However, there is a contingent that has been trained by others who have been trained to say, without evidence, that vitamin and mineral supplements are harmful. This misinformation has been repeated so often by these people that they believe it. If their intent is to warn about abuse or to remind everyone that there is an upper limit of safety, fine. But their warnings should be rephrased to emphasize not taking too much rather than not taking any at all.

Vitamin and mineral supplements have been used for fifty years with a safety history greater than that of any other food product or medication. Yes, far more people die of strangulation on hot dogs or allergic reaction to peanuts than experience side effects from supplements. No death has ever been reported from self-administration of vitamin supplements.

But how many times have you heard some "authority" claim that there are "more than 4,000 cases of vitamin poisonings each year"? The word "poison" implies grave illness or death to most people. In fifty years of vitamin supplementation there has never been a vitamin-caused fatality reported in an adult in the U.S., while each of the following *has* caused disability and death: peanuts, strawberries, rhubarb, under-cooked pork, broad beans, and shellfish. Nor has there been a report of a death of a child due to the accidental consumption of a jar of vitamins.

Yes, iron, vitamin A, vitamin D, and several trace minerals can be toxic and lead to death. The only reported cases are arctic explorers eating polar bear liver, which concentrates and stores large amounts of vitamin A, and children during World War II who, when vitamin drops for infants became available, were mistakenly given teaspoon amounts instead of drop amounts. Iron toxicity has caused problems in children, and that is why supplements containing iron have child-proof caps though they are formulated for children.

When *Supernutrition: Megavitamin Therapy* was published in 1975 there were dire predictions of disaster. However, all that happened was that the nation's health improved and I received thousands of thank-you letters and "God blesses," which made my efforts worthwhile. According to those who wrote to me, hundreds of lives were saved and thousands of people were helped to enjoy a better life.

Since then other researchers and physicians have published books about their successful programs that made my supplement recommendations, so shocking in 1975, look puny by comparison. The Supernutrition amounts are, in fact, moderate; but more important, they are *optimal*.

The vitamin poisoning myth was first brought to my attention in 1977 by the famous writer of inspirational books Marjorie Holmes. She was researching for her outstanding book *God and Vitamins,* and after one of my lectures at a Washington, D.C.–area university she asked me why the FDA would say that vitamins cause thousands of poisonings each year. We set out together to track down the source of misinformation, but it was Marjorie Holmes who got to the bottom of the myth.

The problem began with the March, 1974 issue of the *FDA Consumer,* published monthly by the FDA. At times, and especially during the 1970s, this publication has served to propagandize against the use of vitamin supplements, and it has been found to be deficient in terms of balance and verification of statements. The FDA then reprinted this story as a pamphlet called "Myths of Vitamins." The pamphlet has since omitted the error, but it was etched in the minds of some forever.

The 1974 *FDA Consumer* article misquoted an article from the April–June 1972 "National Clearinghouse for Poison Control Centers Bulletin" by George D. Armstrong. The Armstrong article is entitled "Vitamin Ingestions." Yes, the article was about vitamin *ingestions*, not vitamin poisonings! The article mentioned vitamin ingestion reports thirty times and only used the word "poisoning" five times to describe the nineteen attempts at *self-poisoning* (gestures of suicide or suicide attempts—but no chance, try something else) or to explain that vitamin A poisoning could only normally occur at high dosages over a long period of time.

For the *FDA Consumer* article to refer to vitamin ingestions as poisonings was a gross misrepresentation of the "Poison Control Centers Bulletin." There is a vast difference between a report of a mother taking a child to a health care facility because her child ate a whole bottle of vitamins and she is worried, and an actual serious illness caused by a poisonous compound. Yet the *FDA Consumer* and "Myths of Vitamins" have been quoted as gospel by physicians and dieticians for two decades. Just as you can't un-ring a bell, you can't stop the repetition of this ridiculous myth. Many have tried to get the FDA to send out a correction, but the best that they would do was to omit the statement in later reprinting.

The 1972 Armstrong article was very clear that there were no serious problems. In fact, because there were so many accidental ingestion reports and so few illnesses, one can only conclude that vitamins are very safe. The Armstrong article begins, "Over the past several years, vitamins have been exceeded only by aspirin in the number of ingestions reported to the clearinghouse. . . . Public and medical knowledge of the relative safety of vitamins probably results in a laxity in reporting ingestions."

For the 4,000 vitamin ingestions reported, *only forty-five people were hospitalized (mostly for observation), and there were no fatalities!* The report states, "In the 1,971 reported cases involving children that were treated, 908 of the 1,030 treated cases had no symptoms. There were 58 cases having nausea, vomiting, and/or abdominal pain. Twelve children exhibited lethargy, two rashes, two pneumonias, two elevated temperatures, and one ataxia."

Yet the poisoning myth was still propagated by the March 1984 *FDA Consumer.* An article entitled "Vitamins, Aspirin Lead Poisonings" begins with a statement that vitamins and baby aspirin "are the most frequently mentioned causes of accidental *poisonings* in children under the age of five." After identifying vitamins as a poison, the article states that there were well over 745,000 cases of poisonings in the under-five age group in 1980. This would lead one to conclude that most of the 745,000 reported ingestions were of vitamins. Then the second paragraph states, "Childhood poisoning continues to pose a major public health problem in the United States. An estimated fifty to eighty youngsters still die every year as a result of ingesting harmful substances."

At this point in the article only two specific products—vitamins and aspirin—have been mentioned. Both are identified as poisons, and then fifty to eighty deaths in children due to poisonings are mentioned. Nowhere is it mentioned that vitamins are not acute poisons. Nowhere is the actual number of reported vitamin ingestions listed. Nowhere is the reader told that there were no deaths due to vitamin ingestions. Of course, aspirin causes deaths nearly every year. But the FDA doesn't pick on aspirin—only vitamins, for some reason.

The figures for 1983 show that there are an estimated 2.3 million so-called "poisonings" each year, of which 251,012 were documented by the American Association of Poison Control Centers. The AAPCC represents sixteen poison control centers serving 11% of the U.S. population. The reported poisonings resulted in ninety-five deaths. Of those deaths, more than half were suicides. Vitamins caused no deaths!

Of the 251,012 reported poisonings, three fifths (150,857) involved over-the-counter drugs and prescriptions. Of these, painkillers such as aspirin and acetaminophen accounted for 25,771 poisonings leading to 22 deaths. Sedatives, sleep aids, and tranquilizers caused 8,487 poisonings and eleven deaths. Vitamins caused no deaths.

Cleaning agents caused 22,347 poisonings leading to four deaths. Pesticides caused 8,438 poisonings and four deaths. Cosmetics caused 13,192 poisonings and two deaths. Alcohol caused 9,201 poisonings in children under six years of age, which resulted in twelve deaths. Eating plant leaves caused 22,326 poisonings and no deaths. Vitamins caused no deaths.

Keep in mind that these reported poisonings with ingestions of things such as plant leaves or vitamins are not usually poisonings, but worried parents rush the kids to a hospital because Johnnie ate a leaf off of a bush.

Now, the Food and Drug Administration has proved the safety of vitamin and mineral supplements. They didn't set out to do so, but they did prove it.

In early 1986 the American Dietetic Association had been involved in two press conferences to warn the public about possibly "poisoning themselves with megadoses of vitamins and minerals." No cases could be cited, just general, unfounded warnings. However, these headlines prompted the FDA to monitor closely persons taking food supplements for adverse health effects.

An FDA spokesman at these conferences, Dr. Allan Forbes, director of Nutrition and Food Sciences, was quoted as saying, "Americans may be poisoning themselves with megadoses of vitamins and minerals, potentially causing problems related to the very ones they are trying to prevent. . . . My great hope is that we'll build an increasing body of study on toxicity, but until the data base is adequate, we can't do it [regulate]. . . . We're looking for clear documentation of toxicity associated with vitamin and mineral use to help us with the regulatory process. We urge physicians across the United States to join with us in this important effort."

How do you like your crow served, Dr. Forbes—broiled with sprouts and oat bran? It has been three years at this writing, and obviously the data base isn't adequate (that is, it doesn't show what he thought it would, so he won't say anything about it and hopes everyone forgets about it).

The FDA called upon all physicians to use the regular drug reporting system for adverse reactions (FDA form 1639a, developed in May 1985). Under the Freedom of Information Act of U.S. Code 552 I obtained all the data collected by the FDA on adverse reactions to drugs, vitamins, minerals, and herbs.

The FDA admits in its publication, *FDA Consumer* (June 1989), that the FDA receives more than 50,000 written reports of adverse drug reactions each year. When requested for information on drug use resulting in death as an adverse reaction, the FDA computer printout of data was 1,696 pages.

As to vitamins, minerals, and herbs, no datum implicated a death was due to misuse, overuse, or accidental ingestion of any vitamin, mineral, or herb. There were a few reports of death from various causes in which the persons were taking vitamins along with drugs, but there was no suggestion that the vitamins were harmful in any way.

As an example, there were fourteen reports involving, among other things, folic acid, with one of those reports describing a patient who had died. This patient had a congenital anomaly and epilepsy and was also taking dilantin, phenobarbital, and tegretol.

Another report mentioned radiation sickness in a cancer patient who was taking fluorouracil. You get the picture. Folic acid has no known side effects, whereas the drug and other treatment have the side effects reported.

In similar reports, vitamin A was included four times, with no deaths involved. One example is a congenital anomaly in a DES daughter. The ability of DES to cause birth defects is widely known.

Vitamin E was reported twice, once in a patient having a fever, and once in a patient who died. The latter was a cancer patient who was also taking chemotherapy. The fever patient was also taking thiopental, nitrous oxide, and halothane.

Vitamin K was reported four times, and "vitamins" five times. The complaints included headache, nausea, abortion, gastrointestinal bleed, and ulcers, but no deaths. Of course, the patients were taking drugs for other conditions and were not taking vitamins alone.

A grand total of twenty-nine unfounded complaints out of 150,000 over three years is not bad. Thank you, FDA, for clarifying the made-up issue of food supplement safety.

The subject has been reviewed in the literature many times. The evidence shows that vitamin C as commonly used in megavitamin doses does not cause kidney stones or abortions. Selenium is not toxic in the range needed for protection from cancer, which is the RDA. Vitamin E does not make you tired but actually energizes most people.

However, as with everything else, there is a safety limit. You should not exceed what has been shown to be safe through many years unless you are doing so under the care of a health professional. And there are individuals with certain genetic defects who shouldn't take too much iron—but these individuals should have been identified in their first years of life. There are others who may be sensitive to lower levels of nutrients than normal, but the Supernutrition ranges are conservative enough for even these unique individuals.

The next chapter discusses the ranges of nutrients that produce optimal health.

27

The New Supernutrition
Plan

The official Recommended Dietary Allowances (RDAs) are not intended to be the *optimal* amounts of nutrients for *optimal* health. The New Supernutrition Plan is closer to the optimal level, and when modified with the specific suggestions given in each chapter in this book as needed, your optimal dietary intake is obtained.

The "official" RDAs are set by a subcommittee of the Food and Nutrition Board of the National Research Council of the National Academy of Sciences. Page eight of the tenth edition states, "RDAs are neither minimal requirements nor necessarily optimal levels of intake."[1] I concur 100%! "RDAs are safe and adequate levels reflecting the state of knowledge concerning a nutrient, its bioavailability, and variations among the U.S. population." The correctness of this statement depends on the interpretation of "adequate."

The RDAs are intended to keep genetically typical, healthy persons in average health. To me that is not adequate. Average health is unacceptable unless you are in below-average health. The goal of this book is SUPER HEALTH or optimal

TABLE 27.1
Food and Nutrition Board, National Academy of Sciences—National Research Council Recommended Dietary Allowances,[a] Revised 1989

Designed for the maintenance of good nutrition of practically all healthy people in the United States

Category	Age (years) or Condition	Weight (kg)	Weight (lb)	Height (cm)	Height (in)	Protein (g)	Fat-soluble Vitamins: Vita-min A (μg RE)[c]	Vita-min D (μg)[d]	Vita-min E (mgα-TE)[e]	Vita-min K (μg)
Infants	0.0–0.5	6	13	60	24	13	375	7.5	3	5
	0.5–1.0	9	20	71	28	14	375	10	4	10
Children	1–3	13	29	90	35	16	400	10	6	15
	4–6	20	44	112	44	24	500	10	7	20
	7–10	28	62	132	52	28	700	10	7	30
Males	11–14	45	99	157	62	45	1,000	10	10	45
	15–18	66	145	176	69	59	1,000	10	10	65
	19–24	72	160	177	70	58	1,000	10	10	70
	25–50	79	174	176	70	63	1,000	5	10	80
	51+	77	170	173	68	63	1,000	5	10	80
Females	11–14	46	101	157	62	46	800	10	8	45
	15–18	55	120	163	64	44	800	10	8	55
	19–24	58	128	164	65	46	800	10	8	60
	25–50	63	138	163	64	50	800	5	8	65
	51+	65	143	160	63	50	800	5	8	65

Pregnant	60	800	10	10	65
Lactating 1st 6 months	65	1,300	10	12	65
2nd 6 months	62	1,200	10	11	65

ᵃThe allowances, expressed as average daily intakes over time, are intended to provide for individual variations among most normal persons as they live in the United States under usual environmental stresses. Diets should be based on a variety of common foods in order to provide other nutrients for which human requirements have been less well defined. See text for detailed discussion of allowances and of nutrients not tabulated.

ᵇWeights and heights of Reference Adults are actual medians for the U.S. population of the designated age, as reported by NHANES II. The median weights and heights of those under 19 years of age were taken from Hamill et al. (1979) (see pages 16–17). The use of these figures does not imply that the height-to-weight ratios are ideal.

ᶜRetinol equivalents. 1 retinol equivalent = 1 μg retinol or 6 μg β-carotene. See text for calculation of vitamin A activity of diets as retinol equivalents.

ᵈAs cholecalciferol. 10 μg cholecalciferol = 400 IU of vitamin D.

ᵉα-tocopherol equivalents. 1 mg d-α tocopherol = 1 α-TE. See text for variation in allowances and calculation of vitamin E activity of the diet as α-tocopherol equivalents.

Reprinted from Reference 1

TABLE 27.1 (continued)

Food and Nutrition Board, National Academy of Sciences—
National Research Council Recommended Dietary Allowances,[a] Revised 1989

Designed for the maintenance of good nutrition of practically all healthy people in the United States

Category	Age (years) or Condition	Weight[b] (kg)	(lb)	Height[b] (cm)	(in)	Water-Soluble Vitamins Vitamin C (mg)	Thiamine (mg)	Riboflavin (mg)	Niacin (mg NE)[f]	Vitamin B-6 (mg)	Folate (µg)	Vitamin B-12 (µg)
Infants	0.0-0.5	6	13	60	24	30	0.3	0.4	5	0.3	25	0.3
	0.5-1.0	9	20	71	28	35	0.4	0.5	6	0.6	35	0.5
Children	1-3	13	29	90	35	40	0.7	0.8	9	1.0	50	0.7
	4-6	20	44	112	44	45	0.9	1.1	12	1.1	75	1.0
	7-10	28	62	132	52	45	1.0	1.2	13	1.4	100	1.4
Males	11-14	45	99	157	62	50	1.3	1.5	17	1.7	150	2.0
	15-18	66	145	176	69	60	1.5	1.8	20	2.0	200	2.0
	19-24	72	160	177	70	60	1.5	1.7	19	2.0	200	2.0
	25-50	79	174	176	70	60	1.5	1.7	19	2.0	200	2.0
	51+	77	170	173	68	60	1.2	1.4	15	2.0	200	2.0
Females	11-14	46	101	157	62	50	1.1	1.3	15	1.4	150	2.0
	15-18	55	120	163	64	60	1.1	1.3	15	1.5	180	2.0
	19-24	58	128	164	65	60	1.1	1.3	15	1.6	180	2.0
	25-50	63	138	163	64	60	1.1	1.3	15	1.6	180	2.0
	51+	65	143	160	63	60	1.0	1.2	13	1.6	180	2.0

Pregnant	70	1.5	1.6	17	2.2	400	2.2
Lactating 1st 6 months	95	1.6	1.8	20	2.1	280	2.6
2nd 6 months	90	1.6	1.7	20	2.1	260	2.6

a The allowances, expressed as average daily intakes over time, are intended to provide for individual variations among most normal persons as they live in the United States under usual environmental stresses. Diets should be based on a variety of common foods in order to provide other nutrients for which human requirements have been less well defined. See text for detailed discussion of allowances and of nutrients not tabulated.

b Weights and heights of Reference Adults are actual medians for the U.S. population of the designated age, as reported by NHANES II. The median weights and heights of those under 19 years of age were taken from Hamill et al. (1979) (see pages 16—17). The use of these figures does not imply that the height-to-weight ratios are ideal.

c 1 NE (niacin equivalent) is equal to 1 mg of niacin or 60 mg of dietary tryptophan.

Reprinted from Reference 1

TABLE 27.1 (continued)
Food and Nutrition Board, National Academy of Sciences—National Research Council Recommended Dietary Allowances,[a] Revised 1989
Designed for the maintenance of good nutrition of practically all healthy people in the United States

Category	Age (years) or Condition	Weight[b] (kg)	Weight[b] (lb)	Height[b] (cm)	Height[b] (in)	Calcium (mg)	Phosphorus (mg)	Magnesium (mg)	Iron (mg)	Zinc (mg)	Iodine (µg)	Selenium (µg)
Infants	0.0–0.5	6	13	60	24	400	300	40	6	5	40	10
	0.5–1.0	9	20	71	28	600	500	60	10	5	50	15
Children	1–3	13	29	90	35	800	800	80	10	10	70	20
	4–6	20	44	112	44	800	800	120	10	10	90	20
	7–10	28	62	132	52	800	800	170	10	10	120	30
Males	11–14	45	99	157	62	1,200	1,200	270	12	15	150	40
	15–18	66	145	176	69	1,200	1,200	400	12	15	150	50
	19–24	72	160	177	70	1,200	1,200	350	10	15	150	70
	25–50	79	174	176	70	800	800	350	10	15	150	70
	51+	77	170	173	68	800	800	350	10	15	150	70
Females	11–14	46	101	157	62	1,200	1,200	280	15	12	150	45
	15–18	55	120	163	64	1,200	1,200	300	15	12	150	50
	19–24	58	128	164	65	1,200	1,200	280	15	12	150	55
	25–50	63	138	163	64	800	800	280	15	12	150	55
	51+	65	143	160	63	800	800	280	10	12	150	55

Pregnant	1,200	1,200	320	30	15	175	65
Lactating 1st 6 months	1,200	1,200	355	15	19	200	75
2nd 6 months	1,200	1,200	340	15	16	200	75

a The allowances, expressed as average daily intakes over time, are intended to provide for individual variations among most normal persons as they live in the United States under usual environmental stresses. Diets should be based on a variety of common foods in order to provide other nutrients for which human requirements have been less well defined. See text for detailed discussion of allowances and of nutrients not tabulated.

b Weights and heights of Reference Adults are actual medians for the U.S. population of the designated age, as reported by NHANES II. The median weights and heights of those under 19 years of age were taken from Hamill et al. (1979) (see pages 16–17). The use of these figures does not imply that the height-to-weight ratios are ideal.

Reprinted from Reference 1

health. Average health means three to four colds a year, the flu every year or two, a major operation every decade, and unacceptable risk of heart disease and cancer at too young an age.

Now, we can't live forever, and we are all human, and even with SUPER HEALTH we will get a cold every five years or so, and the flu every ten years or so, and a major operation once in our lifetime, and eventually we will get a fatal ailment. The goal of SUPER HEALTH is not to get the fatal illnesses until well beyond the average lifespan and not to pass away until we approach the maximum human lifespan. But SUPER HEALTH is more than being free from disease—it's being so healthy that you burst with energy, your body is strong, and your mind is sharp. *SUPER HEALTH is living better longer and living all the days of our lives.*

Table 27.1 lists the 1989 RDAs as published in the tenth edition of the Recommended Dietary Allowances.

The RDAs are divided into ten age groups, plus three categories for pregnant and lactating women. The RDAs for adults include separate groupings for men and women, although the differences are few except for weight, calorie intake, calcium, and iron.

The first distinction between the RDAs and the New Supernutrition Plan is that there is no category for either pregnant or lactating women. That is a matter that should be closely monitored by the woman's personal physician. If the woman is not under the close supervision of her family physician, obstetrician, or pediatrician, which would be extremely unfortunate, the woman should rely on the RDAs.

The second distinction is that the New Supernutrition Plan is not based on age or sex. It is based on diet, health status, and life-style. The New Supernutrition Plan is not intended for infants or children. It is intended for intelligent adults who want to get the most out of their lives. There are four basic categories based on diet, health status, and life-style.

The third distinction is that the New Supernutrition Plan uses safe and optimal ranges rather than one specific value. You can adjust the level to fit what feels best to you, what your supplements provide, and the number of supplements that fits your life-style. The ranges allow for some "overage" to ensure that base levels are achieved while providing a safe and reasonable upper limit.

The fourth distinction is that the basic New Supernutrition Plan is adjusted by the ranges given in applicable chapters to produce your optimal dietary allowances. At the risk of repeating myself, I want to be clear in stating that these various contributions to your optimal dietary allowances—the basic New Supernutrition Plan and the ranges indicated in applicable chapters—*are not additive*. You are to use the highest range for a given nutrient. You are not to add all of the ranges for each nutrient together.

The fifth distinction is that the tables list *supplementation level, not total dietary intake*. You don't have to try and calculate your daily dietary intake, as that is already considered in the various categories. The table values represent suggested supplementation ranges for your consideration.

Table 27.2 lists the basic New Supernutrition Plan values. There are four basic categories:

- Category A—Persons who have excellent diets, are very active or exercise regularly, are of good health, are near ideal weight, and have no family history of premature illness or premature death.
- Category B—Persons who have good diets, are fairly active, have average health, have normal blood pressure, and are not obese.
- Category C—Persons with average diets, little physical activity, and poorer than average health.
- Category D—Persons with poor diets *or* poor health *or* no exercise and a sedentary life-style.

TABLE 27.2
The Basic New Supernutrition Plan Values

Nutrient	Category A	Category B	Category C	Category D
Vitamins				
A(IU)	5,000–10,000	5,000–10,000	10,000–15,000	10,000–25,000
Beta-carotene (IU)	5,000–10,000	7,500–15,000	10,000–15,000	15,000–25,000
B-1 (mg)	5–10	10–25	25–75	50–100
B-2 (mg)	5–10	10–25	25–75	50–100
B-3 (mg)	25–50	25–75	50–100	75–250
B-6 (mg)	5–25	10–50	25–100	50–100
B-12 (mcg)	5–10	10–25	25–100	50–150
C (mg)	250–2,000	2,000–5,000	2,000–7,500	2,500–12,000
D (IU)	200–400	200–400	300–500	400–1,000
E (IU)	100–200	200–400	400–800	400–1,000
Pantothenic acid (mg)	10–25	25–100	50–250	75–250
Folic acid (mcg)	400–800	400–800	400–800	400–800
Choline (mg)	5–10	10–20	25–100	50–100
Inositol (mg)	5–10	10–20	25–100	50–100
Biotin (mcg)	10–25	15–50	25–100	50–100
PABA (mg)	5–10	5–25	25–100	50–100

Minerals (milligrams, unless otherwise noted)

Selenium (mcg)	50–100	75–200	100–200	150–200
Chromium (mcg)	100–200	100–200	200–300	200–400
Calcium	100–250	100–250	200–400	250–500
Magnesium	75–200	100–300	200–500	250–600
Zinc	5–15	10–25	15–30	20–40
Copper	1–2	1–2	2–3	2–3
Manganese	—	1–5	1–5	1–6
Molybdenum (mcg)	—	25–75	50–150	75–250
Iron	—	5–10	5–15	10–25
Silicon	—	—	15–25	25–90
Potassium	—	—	10–25	50–250
Boron	—	—	1–3	2–4
Iodine (mcg)	—	—	25–150	50–175
Phosphorus	—	—	—	—

Other Food Factors

Pycnogenol	—	—	50–100	100–150
Coenzyme Q-10	—	—	10–30	30–60
Carnitine	—	—	25–100	50–250
Lecithin (caps)	—	—	1–2	1–4
Cysteine	—	—	50–100	100–250
DMG	—	—	50–100	100–150
Taurine	—	—	—	50–100
Tyrosine	—	—	—	50–100

TABLE 27.2 (continued)
The Basic New Supernutrition Plan Values

Nutrient	Category A	Category B	Category C	Category D
Other Food Factors				
Quercetin	—	—	—	100–500
Bromelain	—	—	—	50–200
GLA (caps)	—	—	—	1–2
EPA (caps)	—	—	—	1–4
SOD	—	—	—	—
MPS	—	—	—	—
PAK	—	—	—	—
Garlic	—	—	—	—
Inosine	—	—	—	—
Beta-sitosterol	—	—	—	—
Gamma-oryzanol	—	—	—	—
Octacosanol	—	—	—	—

Appendix

Author's Background

More than thirty years of biochemical and nutritional experience go into this completely rewritten update of the book *Supernutrition: Megavitamin Revolution* that greatly influenced the health of this nation. It started the popular trend toward improving one's health by optimizing one's nourishment.

Richard Passwater's discoveries have led to worldwide recognition. He is listed in *Who's Who in the World, Who's Who in America, American Men and Women of Science,* and *Who's Who in the Frontiers of Science.* Yet he considers his greatest honors his family, his selection as Citizen of the Year in his community, the privilege of being the chief of his community's volunteer fire department, and receiving the nutrition industry's Achievement Award in 1989.

Richard Passwater is a biochemist widely recognized for his health research. His laboratory experience in gerontology, nutrition, and spectroscopy has brought together diverse disciplines resulting in many discoveries, some of which have been patented in more than ten countries.

Richard Passwater is recognized as a leader in free-radical pathology and fluorometry and a foremost expert in trace nutrients in health. He is a student of the scientific literature as well as a laboratory experimenter.

According to Dr. Raymond Chen of the National Institutes of Health, "Passwater marshals much new scientific evidence to support his ideas—few people know the world literature on nutrition and health as well as he."

Nobel Laureate Dr. Linus Pauling stated in *People* magazine (Dec. 15, 1980), "Passwater is reliable, with a good background and knowledge." Dr. Pauling also recommends Richard Passwater's books in his own books.

Nutritionist Dr. Carlton Fredericks wrote, "Richard Passwater is a dedicated, well-qualified biochemist who offers expert, clear guidance in the application of the principles of nutrition for superior health."

Nutrition editor Harald Taub adds, "Richard Passwater is one of a rare breed. There is no nutritional research, no matter how obscure or recent, that Passwater is not aware of or does not take into account."

The author is the director of research at the Solgar Nutritional Research Center in Ocean Pines, Berlin, MD 21811 (USA), a division of Solgar Co., Inc., of Lynbrook, New York 11563 (USA), of which he is also a corporate vice president.

His research emphases are in trace nutrients having antioxidant capability and in isolating unidentified nutrients present in several natural foods but missing in refined synthetic diets containing all the "known" nutrients.

Previously he has been vice president of research for the American Gerontological Research Laboratories, Inc. (Rockville, MD), a division of Life Science Labs, Inc. (Minneapolis, MN); Applications Research Laboratory director for the American Instrument division (Silver Spring, MD) of Baxter-Travenol Laboratories, Inc.; and supervisor of the Instrumental Analyses Laboratory for the Baker and Adamson division (Marcus Hook, PA) of Allied Chemical Corp., Inc.

The author's education includes a B.S. in chemistry from the University of Delaware in 1959 and a Ph.D. in biochemistry from Bernadean University in 1976. At the time of his matriculation at the University of Delaware it was rated the number-two university for chemistry and chemical engineering by *Chemical & Engineering News,* the news magazine of the American Chemical Society. The University of Delaware had been consistently ranked in the top three schools at that time and today is still consistently ranked in the top ten ACS-certified chemistry programs.

He was certified by the American Chemical Society on

August 27, 1959 and has earned "fellow" status in the American Institute of Chemists.

The author's chemical education probably started at the age of eight, when he "commandeered" his brother's chemistry set. Being raised in the "Chemical Capital of the World" and living across from a public library didn't hurt his progress any. Wilmington, Delaware was the home of many chemical firms, including DuPont, Hercules, and Atlas (ICI). He was raised on the banks of the Brandywine River almost directly across from the famous DuPont Experimental Station, the Dupont Co.'s research center. The DuPont family was instrumental in bringing the best possible professors to the University of Delaware.

With a library across the street, the author spent many hours reading his favorite books on chemistry. He understood the high school chemistry textbooks while he was in the eighth grade and had a working knowledge of the college texts when he was in the ninth grade.

He chose Bernadean University because it offered a program in naturopathy as well as biochemistry, was a "university without walls" having an outreach program to provide instructors in various locations, and allowed partial credit for published scientific papers and work experience. This program allowed the author to continue his education while still being able to conduct his research and support his family.

His dissertation was "Dietary Influences on the Alternative Metabolic Pathways of Cholesterol." At the time of his enrollment at Bernadean University it was accredited by the International Commission for the Accreditation of Colleges and Universities, Ltd. The pioneering program offered by Bernadean University was ahead of its time, and without state or government grants they had to close their doors in 1981.

He is also a graduate of the University of Maryland Fire and Rescue Institute and the Maryland Institute for Emergency Medical Services Systems. He has been the fire chief of the Ocean Pines Volunteer Fire Department since 1984 and is an emergency medical technician and a volunteer for the Worcester County Health Department. He holds the highest levels of achievement recognized by Maryland, Firefighter III and Advanced Rescue Technician. He is the chairman of the Worcester County Emergency Planning Committee (LEPC).

The author is past vice president of the International Foundation for Preventive Medicine, Inc. (1977–81), past president of the American Academy of Applied Health Sciences (1982–4), and past president of Sub-Aqueous Exploration, Inc. (1983–4). He was the Washington representative for the Institute of Nutritional Research (1975–9) and past lecturer for the Donsbach University outreach program (1978–84).

The author was a founding member and serves on the board of directors of the Worcester Memorial Hospital, which oversees the operation of Atlantic General Hospital. He has served on the board of directors of the Ocean Pines Volunteer Fire Department since 1981. He is a member of the board of advisors to the National Institute of Nutritional Education, the Coalition for Alternatives in Nutrition and Healthcare, Inc., and the International Academy of Holistic Health and a past member of the board of directors of the International Foundation for Preventive Medicine, Inc. (1977–81) and the Worcester County School Board Advisory Committee (1983–4). He formerly served as a member of the board of directors of Life Science Labs, Inc., Scientific Documentation Center, Ltd., and Sub-Aqueous Exploration, Inc.

Richard Passwater serves on the editorial boards of "Whole Foods" and "VIM Newsletter." He is a health columnist for "Whole Foods" and a past columnist for "Your Good Health." In the past he has been editor of *Fluorescence News,* on the editorial board of *Analytical Letters,* and a reviewer for *Analytical Chemistry.* He has served on the editorial boards of the *Journal of Holistic Medicine,* the official journal of the American Holistic Medical Association, and *Nutritional Perspectives.*

Also included in the scientific societies to which he belongs are the American Aging Association, American Association for the Advancement of Science, American Chemical Society (certified 1959), American Geriatrics Society, American Institute of Chemists (elected Fellow, 1985), American Society for Preventive Dentistry, Chemical Society of Washington, International Academy of Holistic Health and Medicine, International Academy of Preventive Medicine, International Foundation for Preventive Medicine, International

Union of Pure and Applied Chemistry, New York Academy of Science, Nutrition Today Society, Royal Society of Chemistry (London), and Society for Applied Spectroscopy.

The author has chaired sections of national and regional scientific symposia, including the 1970 National Society of Applied Spectroscopy Meeting, Symposium on Advances in Spectroscopy Instrumentation, New Orleans, October 1970, and the Symposium on Fluorescence, University of Maryland, February 1967.

He currently is a liaison to Congress for the American Chemical Society's Department of Government Relations and Science Policy.

The author has published dozens of articles in the scientific literature on the aging process, cancer, cholesterol, selenium, dieting, and fluorometry. A few representative selections are "Energy Transfer between Isoalloxazines and Phenothiazines" [*Journal of Luminescence* 1(2):470–480 (1970)], "Plans for a Large Scale Study of Possible Retardation of the Human Aging Process" [*The Gerontologist* 10(3):11, 28 (1970)], "Protein Missyntheses" [*Chemical and Engineering News* 9–10) May 10, 1971)], "Physics of the Cell Membrane [a five-part series in *American Laboratory* 6(4):59–74 (1974), 6(6):19–29 (1974), 6(11):49–62 (1974), 7(1):41–50 (1975), 8(4):37–47 (1976)], "Cancer: New Directions" [*American Laboratory* 4(9):23–35 (1972)], "Function of Vitamin E" [*Chemical and Engineering News* 53 (October 9, 1972)], "Dietary Cholesterol" [*American Laboratory* 4(9):23–35 (1972)], "Human Aging Research" [*American Laboratory* 3(4):36–40 (1971) and 3(5):21–26(1971)], "War on Malnutrition" [*Chemical and Engineering News* 41 (Jan. 11, 1971)], and "Antioxidant Protection" [*Chemical and Engineering News* 3 (Oct. 28, 1974)].

Chemical Abstracts and *ISI Citation References* provide further details. Abstracts of his journal articles are found in *Chemical Abstracts* as 84(25)177692n, 83(9)74099z, 83(8)68960g, 83(7)56755f, 83(5)41838m, 82(19)120487d, 82(15)96507n, 82(10)67644z, 81(15)87268n, 81(3)10504d, 79(20)119913w, 79(11)64106c, 79(5)29120f, 77(21)138609b, 77(13)86000z, 77(11)73131t, 77(3)15076t, 75(6)44454d, 74(5)19620b, 73(16)85824f, and 71(25)121863h. (A detailed list of publications is available upon request.)

Abstracts of his patents are included in *Chemical Ab-*

stracts as 80(21)119314x and 77(26)168633x.

Abstracts of his books are included in *Chemical Abstracts* as 99(13)104217, 84(13)88479f, 82(20)132021k, 74(8)36856a, and 67(4)16673r.

His technical books include *Guide to Fluorescence Literature* [Plenum Press, vol. 1 (1967), vol. 2 (1970), and vol. 3 (1974)]. This highly praised three-volume, 15,000-reference guide is warmly referred to as "The Passwater" in scientific journals [*J. Opt. Soc. Am.* (May 1971)].

The author's previous books for general audiences are described later.

As a service to the scientific community, the author was a volunteer abstractor for *Chemical Abstracts* from 1960 through 1966.

The author holds several international patents on formulations to prevent and treat cancer, and one on formulations for life extension. These patents, based on antioxidant nutrients, were filed starting in 1970 and today are the subject of research by the National Cancer Institute and other agencies. Human clinical trials confirming important parts of Richard Passwater's early animal studies have recently been published. (See "Synergistic effect of vitamin E and selenium in the chemoprevention of mammary carcinogenesis," Horvath, P. M., and Ip, C., *Cancer Research* 43:5335–41, Nov. 1983; "Prediagnostic serum selenium and risk of cancer," Willet, W. C., et al., *Lancet,* 130–4, July 16, 1983; and "Plasma retinol, beta-carotene and vitamin E levels in relation to the future risk of breast cancer," Wald, N. J., et al., *British Journal of Cancer* 49:321–4, 1984.)

A summary of the patents and continuing patent applications follows: United States—39140, 97011, 271655, 398596, 481788, 593812, 613420, 718469, 806534, 930657; Australia—29107/71; Belgium—767442; Canada—142747; Denmark—2432/71; France—71-18380, 73-27942; Germany—P-21-24-972,9, P-23-36-17 6.4; Great Britain—16047/71, 34785/73, 1444024; Mexico—127400; Netherlands—71.06929; New Zealand—163719; and Sweden—6520/71.

Besides his discoveries in cancer and aging research, the author has contributed new concepts to nutritional science, including the Supernutrition principle of optimal nourishment and the FLAB concept of using FLAB units and the FLAB index to better measure the effects of food on body chemistry. Current research by others confirms the FLAB units and index principles that different foods produce insulin responses quite different than that predicted by the previous teachings merely utilizing food composition tables in regard to carbohydrate type and protein and fat content. [See P. Capro and J. Olefsky, *New Eng. J. Med.* 309(1):44–45 (July 7, 1983).]

Other important research projects include a joint five-year study with Dr. Linus Pauling (Linus Pauling Institute) and Dr. James Enstrom (UCLA School of Public Health) of the benefits of vitamin supplements on a large group of California volunteers and a study of the protective effect of vitamin E against heart disease. The Enstrom-Pauling study showed that the supplemented volunteers had only two-thirds the death rate expected for typical Californians of the same age, sex, race, etc. [*Proc. Natl. Acad. Sci.* 79, 6023–7 (1982)]. The vitamin E study was a retrospective study of vitamin E users that showed that long-term vitamin E users had less than half of the heart disease rate of typical Americans of the same age, sex, and race (*Prevention,* Jan.–Aug. 1978).

The author's current laboratory research includes the effect of dietary glucose tolerance factor on diabetic (C57BL/KsJ) mice, selenium protection against free-radical-generated cancer in (AKR/J) mice, effect of L-lysine on viral-induced mammary carcinoma in C3H/HeJ mice (jointly with Dr. Christopher Kagan of the Kaiser-Permanente group in Berkeley, CA), isolation of growth factor G, effect of fluoride on 2-FAA-induced cancer in (AKR/J) mice and spontaneous cancer in C3H/HeJ mice. He also studies the role of amino acids in controlling cocaine addiction and environmental pollution.

Prior to entering gerontological and nutritional research the author was one of the world's foremost authorities on fluorometry. As Research Applications Laboratory director at Baxter-Travenol Laboratories (Aminco Division) he developed new procedures for biochemical analyses, extended analytical sensitivity for existing methods, and improved instrumentation design. He developed courses in fluorometry and taught scientists, including Nobel Prize winners, new techniques in analytical instrumentation to extend their research. Students included noted researchers from the National Institutes of Health, leading universities, the Food and

Drug Administration, the Environmental Protection Agency, and industry.

In 1963 the author helped design quality-control procedures for, and participated in, the first large-scale production of liquid hydrogen (U.S. code-named "Project Poppa Bear") for Sterns-Rogers near West Palm Beach, Florida. He also participated in the test-firing of the engine for the Centaur at Pratt-Whitney, the first liquid hydrogen/liquid oxygen–fueled rocket, which was the precursor to the Saturn rocket.

When illicit drug problems escalated in the mid-1960s the author developed methods for urinalysis screening and street detection (Udenfriend, *Fluor. Assay in Biology Med.*, Academic Press, 1960; Guilbault, *Pract. Fluor.*, Dekker, CA 1973). He has worked with several government agencies in setting up screening laboratories. In the early 1970s he assisted the U.S. armed forces in developing screening procedures and contract laboratory certification for detecting illicit drugs in service personnel (*Fluor. News* 6:3, 8–11, 1971). Along with Dr. Leo Goldbaum of the U.S. Army's Walter Reed Hospital Toxicology Laboratory, he developed gas chromatographic screening tests for illicit drug and medicinal drug detection in medical emergencies. He has developed forensic science and criminology methods (*Facts & Methods* 6:2–13, 1965).

The author is currently studying an effective means of controlling the depression and insomnia that follow cocaine withdrawal (problems that are normally solved by the patients' resumption of their cocaine habit) with the amino acids L-tyrosine and L-tryptophan.

Richard Passwater also supervised the Instrumental Analysis Laboratory at General Chemical Corp. and developed special pesticide detection methods.

The author has been twice honored by the Committee for World Health for his "Outstanding Research" (1978 & 1980). In 1976 he was a recipient of a Notable Americans Award. In 1973 he was a nominee for the American Chemical Society's Award in Chemical Education. In 1987 he received the Citizen of the Year Award in his hometown of Ocean Pines, MD for his community service. In 1989 he was awarded the nutrition industry's Achievement Award by *Whole Foods* magazine.

One of his books was chosen by *Library Journal* as one of the top six health books for 1983 and one of the top one hundred science and technology books in a field of 40,000 books [*Trace Elements, Hair Analysis and Nutrition* (with Dr. E. Cranton)].

He has been listed in *Who's Who in the World* since 1984, *Who's Who in America* since 1988, and *Who's Who in the East* since 1977, as well as being included in *American Men and Women of Science, Who's Who in Frontiers of Science and Technology* (second edition, 1985), *Men of Achievement* (7th ed.), *International Registry of Profiles* (1980), *Contemporary Authors* (97–100), *Personalities of America* (1981), and *International Who's Who of Intellectuals* (1981).

He has been an invited lecturer from Russia to Australia and is a member of the International Platform Association.

POPULAR BOOKS, ARTICLES, AND RADIO BROADCASTS

Dr. Passwater has authored several best-selling books, including *Trace Elements, Hair Analysis and Nutrition* (with Elmer Cranton, M.D.) [Keats, 1983], *Selenium as Food and Medicine* (Keats, 1980), *The Easy No-Flab Diet* (Marek, 1979), *Cancer and Its Nutritional Therapies* (Keats, 1978), *Super Calorie, Carbohydrate Counter* (Dale, 1978), *Supernutrition for Healthy Hearts* (Dial Press, 1977; Jove, 1978), *Supernutrition: Megavitamin Revolution* (Dial Press, 1975; Pocket Books, 1976). The author is also the co-editor, with Dr. Earl Mindell, of a series of over fifty "Your Good Health" booklets. He has personally authored the following booklets: "Fish Oils Update" (1987), "Selenium Update" (1986), "Antioxidant Nutrients" (1985), "Beta-carotene" (1984), "Beginners' Vitamin Guide" (1983), "EPA-Marine Lipids" (1982), "GTF-Chromium" (1982), and "Evening Primrose Oil" (1981).

His books have been translated into Spanish, French, Dutch, and Japanese.

He has authored more than 250 articles for the general public in *Cosmopolitan, Family Circle, Forum, Prevention, Let's LIVE, Bestways, Health Quarterly,* and others. He is a columnist for *Your Good Health* and *Whole Foods*.

Articles about Richard Passwater and his research have appeared in *People* (Dec. 1980), *Reader's Digest, Woman's*

*Day, Ladies' Home Journal, Town and Country, National
Enquirer, National Star, Prevention, Let's LIVE, Forum,
Body Forum, SOMA, World Weekly News, National Medical
Examiner,* and others.

He broadcast a nutrition message three times daily on
WMCA in New York. He made more than 7,000 broadcasts
from 1979 to 1986. During 1985–6 he also broadcast a daily
nutritional message series on WNEW in New York. His
broadcasts were carried by station WRNG in Atlanta during
1980–83.

The author has appeared on over one hundred television
shows to discuss his research and books. National shows
have included "Good Morning America," "The David Suss-
kind Show," CBN's "USA Today," and the syndicated "Joe
Franklin Show."

The son of Stanley Leroy Passwater, Sr. and Mabel Rosetta
King Passwater, Richard was born in Wilmington, Delaware
(USA) on October 13, 1937.

In June of 1964 he married Barbara Gayhart of Not-
tingham, Pennsylvania. They currently live near Ocean City,
Maryland. They have two sons, Richard (1967) and Michael
(1970), a daughter-in-law, Ellen, and grandson Matthew
(1989).

The author's hobbies include photography, nature studies,
wildlife art, subaqueous exploration, and archaeology.

Notes

CHAPTER 1

1. Pauling, Linus; *Vitamin C and the Common Cold,* Freeman and Co., San Francisco (1970)
2. Williams, Roger J.; *You Are Extra-Ordinary,* Pyramid Books, NY (1967)
3. Cheraskin, E., Ringsdorf, W. M. & Brecher, A.; *Psychodietetics,* Stein and Day, NY (1974)
4. Passwater, Richard A.; *Supernutrition: Megavitamin Revolution,* Dial Press, NY (1975)
5. International Conference on Genetic Variation and Nutrition Center for Genetics, Nutrition and Health, Washington, DC (June 1988)
   (Also see American J. Clinical Nutrition 48(6):1497–1516 (Dec. 1988)
6. Schneider, Howard A.; Perspectives in Biology and Medicine 29:392–406 (Spring 1986)

CHAPTER 2

1. Kamath, Savitri K., et al.; J. Amer. Die. Assoc. 86(2) 203–6 (Feb. 1986)
2. Tobias, Alice L. and Van Itallie, Theodore B.; J. Amer. Diet. Assoc. 71(9) 253–7 (Sep. 1977)
3. Teitelman, Robert; Forbes 156–7 (Apr. 9, 1984)
4. Bistrian, B. R., et al.; J. Amer. Med. Assoc. 230:858 (1974)
5. Merritt, R. J. and Suskind, R. M.; Amer. J. Clin. Nutr. 32:1320 (1979)

6. Weinsier, R. L., et al.; Amer. J. Clin. Nutr. 32:418 (1979)
7. Nutr. Rev., 46(9)315–7 (1988)

CHAPTER 3

1. Block, Gladys, et al.; Amer. J. Epidemiol. 122(1) 27–40 (1985)
2. *Benefits of Nutritional Supplements*, Council for Responsible Nutrition, Washington, DC (1990)
3. Jolliffe, N.; Metabolism 4:191 (1955)
4. *Science and Education Administration, Nationwide Food Consumption Survey, 1977–78, Preliminary Report No. 2, Food and Nutrient Intakes of Individuals in One Day in the United States*, Spring 1977, U.S. Dept. Agriculture, Washington, D.C. (1980)
5. Anderson, Richard; Amer. J. Clin. Nutr. 41:1177 (June 1985)
6a. Hepburn, F. N.; Amer. J. Clin. Nutr. 35:1297–1301 (1985)
6b. Block, G., et al., Amer. J. Epidemiol. 122:13–26 (1985)
7. J. Nutr. Educ. 12(2) 46–49 (1981)
8. Mareschi, J.-P.; Internat. J. Vit. Nutr. Res. 57:79–85 (1987)
9. *The Food We Eat*, USDA, Misc. Pub. No. 870 (1967)
10. *Protecting Our Food*, USDA Yearbook (1966)
11. Vitamin Communications, Hoffman-LaRoche Inc., Nutley, NJ
12. *Conserving the Nutritive Values in Foods*, USDA, Bul. No. 90 (1965)
13. Schroeder, Henry A.; Amer. J. Clin. Nutr. (May 1971)
14. Bricklin, Mark; *Understanding Vitamins and Minerals*, Rodale Press, Emmaus, PA p16 (1984)
15. Davis, Don. R.; Nutr. Today 16:16–21 1981)
16. *Food*, USDA Yearbook (1959)
17. Lindlahr, Victor H.; *You Are What You Eat*, Newcastle Publ. Co., p42 (1971 ed.)

Also see:

a. Dietary Levels of Households in the United States, Spring 1965, Agriculture Research Service, U.S.D.A., 12–17 (1968)

b. First Health and Nutrition Examination Survey (HANES I), Public Health Service, Health Resources Administration, U.S. Dept. Health (HHS) (1971–2)

c. Rizek, R. L. and Posati, L.; Fam. Econ. Rev. 1:10–17 (1987)

d. Pao, E. M. and Mickle, Sharon J., Food Tech. 24:183 (Sept. 1981)

CHAPTER 4

1. Enstrom, James and Pauling, Linus; Proceed. Nat. Acad. Sci. 79:6023–7 (1982)

2. Enstrom, James; J. Nat. Cancer Inst. 40:356 (Dec. 6, 1989)

3. Breslow, Lester and Belloc, Nedra; Prevent. Med. 1:409–21 (1972)

CHAPTER 5

1. Passwater, Richard A.; 23rd Ann. Mtg. Gerontol. Soc. Toronto (Oct. 21–24, 1970)

2. Passwater, Richard A.; Gerontolog. 10(3) 28(1970)

3. Chem. & Eng. News 48(45) 17 (Oct. 26, 1970)

4. Reuters News Service (Oct. 23, 1970)

5. Prevention 23(12) 104–110 (Dec. 1971)

6. Harman, Denham; J. Gerontol. 23(4) 478 (Oct. 1968)

7. Lemoyne, M., et al.; Amer. J. Clin. Nutr. 46:267–72 (1987)

8. Gohil, K., et al.; J. App. Phys. 63:1638–41 (1987)

9. Packer, L.; Med. Biol. 62:105–9 (1984)

10. Davies, K. J. A., et al.; Biochem. Biophys. Res. Commun. 107:1198–1205 (1982)

11. Bjorksten, Johan and Andrews, Fred; J. Amer. Geriat. Soc. 12(7) 627–631 (July 1964)

12. Tappel, A. L.; in: *Pathological Aspects of Cell Membranes,* Trump, B. F. and Arstila, A. (eds.), Vol. 1, Academic Press, NY (1971)

13. Passwater, Richard A.; Amer. Lab. 5:10–22 (1973)

14. Passwater, Richard A. and Brewer, Keith; Amer. Lab. 8(4) 59–74 (1974)

15. Passwater, Richard A. and Brewer, Keith; Amer. Lab. 6(6) 19–29 (1974)

16. Passwater, Richard A. and Brewer, Keith; Amer. Lab. 6(11) 49–58 (1974)

17. Passwater, Richard A. and Brewer, Keith; Amer. Lab. 7(1) 41–50 (1975)

18. Passwater, Richard A. and Brewer, Keith; Amer. Lab. 8(4) 37–47 (1976)

19. Bliznakov, Emile G.; Aging Dev. 7:189 (1978); also see: Bliznakov, Emile G. and Hunt, G. L.; *The Miracle Nutrient: Coenzyme Q-10* Bantam, NY (1987)

20. Rudman, Daniel, et al.; New Engl. J. Med. 323(1) 1–6 (July 5, 1990)

21. Isidori, A., Lo Monaco, A. and Cappa, M.; Curr. Med. Res. Opin. 7(7) 475–80 (1981)

22. Frei, Balz, England, Laura and Ames, Bruce N.; Proc. Natl. Acad. Sci. 86:6377–6381 (Aug. 1989)

Also see:

Kugler, Hans J.; *Dr. Kugler's Seven Keys to a Longer Life,* Stein & Day, NY (1978)

CHAPTER 6
1. Kuttan, R., et al., Experientia 37:221–3 (1981)

CHAPTER 7
1. Deutch, Stephen I. and Morihisa, John M.; Clin. Neuropharmacol. 11(1)18–35 (1988)

2. Kruck, T. P. A. and McLachlan, D. R. C.; Prog. Clin. Biol. Res. 317:1155–67 (1989)

3. Martyn, C. N., et al., Lancet I (8629):59–62 (Jan. 14, 1989)

4. Ibid., (Feb. 25, 1989)

5. Evans, John R.; Nutr. Rep. 5(12) 89&96 (Dec. 1987)

6. Smith, C. C. T., et al.; J. Neurol. Neurosurg. Psych. v 48 (1985)

7. Burns, A. and Holland, T.; Lancet I:805–6 (1986)

8. Meydani, M., et al.; Nutr. Res. 5:1227–36 (1985)

CHAPTER 8
1. Gerster, H.; Z. Ernahrungswiss 28:56–75 (1989)

2. Taylor, Hugh R., West, Sheila and Emmett, Edward; Wash. Post, A3 (Dec. 1, 1988)

3. Robertson, James McD., Trevithick, J. R. and Donner, Allan P.; Ann. N. Y. Acad. Sci. (In Press 1989) [Also see Sci. News 135:308 (May 20, 1989) and VERIS Special Issue (Feb. 1989)]
4. Trevithick, J. R., et al.; J. Ophthalmol. 16:32–8 (1981)
5. Creighton, M. O., et al.; Exp. Eye Res. 40:213–222 (1985)
6. Stewart-De Haan, P. J., et al.; Exp. Eye Res. 32:54–60 (1981)
7. Creighton, M. O., et al.; Exp. Eye Res. 37:65–76 (1983)
8. Ross, W. M., et al.; J. Ophthalmol. 17:61–66 (1982)
9. Jacques, P., et al.; J. Amer. Coll. Nutr. 6:435 (1987)
10. Jacques, P. F., et al.; Arch. Ophthalmol. 106:337–340 (1988)
11. Nutr. Rev. 47(10) 326–8 (Oct. 1989)

Also see:
   Duarte, Alex; *Cataract Breakthrough,* Internat. Instit. Natural Health Sciences, Huntington Beach, Ca. (1982)

CHAPTER 9

1. Passwater, Richard A.; Prevention 28(7) 66–72 (July 1976)
2. Shute, Wilfrid E. and Taub, Harald J.; *Vitamin E for Ailing & Healthy Hearts,* Pyramid, NY (1972)
3. Shute, Evan; *The Vitamin E Story,* Welch, Ontario (1985)
4. Bergkvist, Leif, et al.; New Eng. J. Med. 321(5) 293–7 (Aug. 3, 1989)

CHAPTER 10

1. Med. World News 42 (Oct. 23, 1989)
2. Wilson, E., Fisher, K. and Fuqua, M.; *Principles of Nutrition,* p144, Wiley, NY (1965)
3. Smith, E. L., et al.; Amer. J. Clin. Nutr. 50:833–42 (1989)
4. Albanese, A. et al.; N.Y. State J. Med. 326 (1975)
5. Dawson-Huges, Bess, et al.; New Eng. J. Med. 323:878–83 (1990)
6. Bullamore, J. et al.; Lancet 2:535–537 (1970)
7. Krook, L. et al.; Cornell Vet. 62:32 (1972)
8. Lutwak, L. et al.; Isrl. J. Med. Sci. 7:504 (1971)

9. British Med. J. (Sep. 24, 1977)
10. Spencer, Herta; Amer. Fam. Phys. 10(2):141 (1974)
11. Spencer, Herta; Ann. Int. Med. (Dec. 1977)
12. Albanese, A.; Dairy Coun. Digest 47(6):34 (Nov.–Dec. 1976)
13. Krook, L.; Cornell Vet 58:59–63 (1968)
14. Horowitz, Michael et al.; Amer. J. Clin. Nutr. 39:857–59 (June 1984)
15. Nielsen, Forrest H., et al.; FASEB J. 1(5) 394–397 (1987)
16. Nielsen, Forrest H., et al.; FASEB J. (Feb. 15, 1989)
17. Carlisle, E. M.; Sci. 167:279–280 (Jan. 16, 1970)
18. Smith, Samuel, et al.; Arch. Intern. Med. 149(11) 2517–9 (1989)

CHAPTER 11

1. Bush, T.; AMA meeting (1974)
2. Lawson, J. and Fischer, P.; Can. Med. J., 55:328 (1951)
3. Champault, Andre; Brit. J. Clin. Pharm. 84:(18) 461–2 (1979)
4. Melman, A., et al.; J. South. Med. Assoc., 73(3):307–309 (1980)
5. Melman, A., et al.; Invest. Urol., 17(6):474–477 (1980)
6. Melman, A., et al.; Invest. Urol., 19(1):46–48 (1981)
7. Melman, A., et al.; J. Urol. (U.S.), 129(3):643–645 (1983)
8. Brown, C. M., et al.; Brit. J. Pharmacol. 66(4) 533–64 (1979)
9. McGrath, J. C.; J. Physiol. 283:23–39 (1978)
10. Jurkiewicz, A. and Jurkiewicz, N. H.; Brit. J. Pharmacol. 56(2) 169–178 (1976)

CHAPTER 12

1. Passwater, Richard A.; Amer. Lab. 5(6) 10–22 (1973)
2. Passwater, Richard A.; U.S. #97011 and others
3. Meydani, S. N. et al.; Mech. Aging and Dev. 34:191–201 (1986)
4. *Diet, Nutrition & Cancer Prevention*, Nat. Instit. Health, Pub. Health Serv., US Dept. HHS, NIH Pub. No. 85-2711 (Nov. 1984)

5. *Diet, Nutrition, and Cancer: Directions for Research*, National Research Council, National Academy Press, Washington, DC (1983)

6. Palmer, Sushma and Bakshi, Kulbir; J. Nat. Can. Inst. 70(6) 1151–1170 (June 1983)

7. Ames, Bruce, et al.; Sci. 221:4617 1256–64 (23 Sep. 1983)

8. Willett, W. C. and MacMahon, B.; New Eng. J. Med. 310(11) 697–703 (15 Mar 1984)

9. Ross, Walter; ACS Cancer News (1982)

10. Ross, Walter; Reader's Digest 78–82 (Feb. 1983)

11. Willett, W. C., et al.; Lancet II:130–4 (July 16, 1983)

12. Yu, Shu-Yu, et al.; Biol. Tr. Elem. Res. 7:21–9 (Jan.–Feb. 1985)

13. Clark, Lawrence C., et al.; Nutr. Cancer 6:13–21 (Jan.–Mar. 1984)

14. Horvath, Paula M. and Ip, Clement; Cancer Res. 43:5335–41 (Nov. 1983)

15. Salonen, J. T., et al.; Brit. Med. J. 290:417–20 (Feb. 9, 1985)

16. Milner, John A.; J. Agric. Food Chem. 32:436–42 (May–June 1984)

17. Kneki, P., et al.; Amer. J. Epidemiol. 127:28–41 (1988)

18. Pothier, Lillian; Cancer 295–303 (Nov. 1, 1987)

19. Shklar, G., et al.; Nutr. Cancer 12:321–325 (1989)

20. Shklar, G., et al.; Nutr. Cancer 12:321–5 (1989)

21. Weisberger, A. and Suhrland, L.; Blood 11:19 (1956)

22. McConnell, K., et al.; J. Nutr. 105:1026–31 (1975)

23. Fex, G., et al.; Nutr. Cancer 10(4) 221–229 (1987)

24. Karmali, R. A., et al.; J. Nat. Cancer Inst. 73:457–61 (Aug. 1984)

25. O'Connor, T. P., et al.; J. Nat. Cancer Inst. 75(5) 959–62 (Nov. 1985)
    (Also see Gabor, H. et al.; J. Nat. Cancer Inst. 75:1223–9 (1986)

26. O'Connor, T. P., Campbell, T. Colin, et al.; J. Nat. Cancer Inst. 81:858–863 (June 7, 1989)

27. Endres, Stefan, et al.; New Engl. J. Med. 320(5) 265–71 (Feb. 2, 1989)

28. The Nutrition Report 3 (August 1989)

29. Corliss, J.; J. Nat. Cancer Inst. 81:1530–1 (Oct. 18, 1989)

30. Gorlin, R.; Arch. Intern. Med. 148: 2043–2048 (1989)
31. Graber, C. D., et al.; J. Infect. Dis. 143(1) 101–5 (Jan. 1981)
32. Reap, Elizabeth A. and Lawson, John W.; J. Lab. Clin. Med. 115:481–6 (1990)

Also see:

Cameron, Ewan and Pauling, Linus; *Cancer and Vitamin C,* Norton and Co., NY (1979)

CHAPTER 13
1. Shekelle, R. B., et al.; Lancet 2:1186–90 (1981)
2. Wald, N., et al.; Lancet 2:813–5 (1980)
3. Kark, J. D., et al.; J. Nat. Cancer Inst. 66:7–16 (1981)
4. Lopez, A. S., et al.; Amer. J. Clin. Nutr. 34:641 (1981)
5. Sprince, Herbert; Private Communication. Also, Executive Health (Jan. 1977)
6. Yonemoto, R. H., Chretien, P. B. and Fehniger, T. F.; Amer. Soc. Clin. Oncology 27:2, 181–192 (1973)
7. Menkes, Marilyn S., et al.; New Eng. J. Med. 315:1250–4 (Nov. 13, 1986)
8. Miyamoto, H., et al.; Cancer 60:1159–62 (1987)
9. Shu-yu, Yu et al.; Biol. Tr. Elem. Res. 24:105–8 (1990)
10. Kneki, P., et al.; Internat. Selenium Conf. (1989)
11. Heimburger, Douglas, et al.; J. Amer. Med. Assoc. 259(10) (March 11, 1988)

Also see:

Cameron, Ewan and Pauling, Linus; *Cancer and Vitamin C,* Norton and Co., NY (1979)

CHAPTER 14
1. Wilkins, T. and Van Tassell, R., eds.; *Human intestinal microflora in health and disease,* Academic Press, NY p265 (1983)
2. Reddy, B. S.; *Dietary fiber in health and disease,* Plenum Press, NY, edited by Vahouny and Kritchevsky p265–62 (1981)
3. Burkitt, D. P.; Cancer 28:3 (1971)
4. Garland, C., et al.; Lancet I:307–9 (Feb. 9, 1985)
5. Lipkin, Martin and Newmark, Harold; N. Engl. J. Med. 313(22) 1381–4 (Nov. 28, 1985)

6. Buset, M., et al.; Cancer Res. 46:5426–30 (Oct. 1986)
7. DeCosse, J.; Nat. Cancer Inst. (Sep. 6, 1989)

CHAPTER 15

1. Shamberger, Raymond and Frost, Douglas; Canad. Med. J. 100:682 (1969)
2. FASEB news briefs; Chem. Eng. News 12 (May 3, 1976)
3. Butterworth, C. E., Jr., et al.; Amer. J. Clin. Nutr. 33:926 (1980)
4. Wald, N. J., et al.; Brit. J. Cancer 49:321–4 (March 1984)
5. Hislop, T. Gregory; Amer. J. Epidemiol. 289 (Feb. 1990)
6. Prentice, F., et al.; J. Nat. Cancer Inst. 124 (Jan. 1990)
7. Chilvers, C., et al.; Lancet 1(8645) 973–82 (May 1989)
8. Whitehead, Nancy, et al.; J. Amer. Med. Assoc. 226:1421–4 (1973)
9. Nutr. Rev. 47(10) 314–7 (Oct. 1989)
10. Brock, K., et al.; Amer. J. Epidem. 124; 518 (1986)
11. Brock, K., et al., J. Nat. Cancer Inst. 80:580–5 (1988)
12. Slattery, M., et al.; Amer. J. Epidem. 130:830 (1989)
13. La Vecchia, C., et al.; Gynecol. Oncol. 30:187–95 (1988)

CHAPTER 16

1. Kok, Frans, et al.; Amer. J. Cardiol. 63:513–6 (1989)
2. Nutr. Rev. 47(8) 247–9 (August 1989)
3. Benditt, Earl P. and Benditt, M. M.; Proc. Nat. Acad. Sci. 70:1753–6 (1973)
4. Henning, B. and Chow, C. K.; Free Radicals in Biology & Medicine 4:99–106 (1988)
5. Phillips, Gerald; Amer. J. Med. 78:363–6 (May 1983)
6. Reaven, Gerald M.; Diabetes 37(12) 1595–1607 (1988)
7. Zavaroni, I.; New Engl. J. Med. 320(11) 702–6 (March 16, 1989)
   Also see New Engl. J. Med. 321(9) 616–8 (1989)
8. Kannel, W. B. et al.; J. Amer. Med. Assoc. (Sep. 4, 1987)
9. J. Amer. Med. Assoc. 251:351–364 (Jan. 20, 1984)
10. New Engl. J. Med. 321:676–600 (1990)
11. [For a rebuttal to Reference #6, see Nutr. Today (March/April 1984)]

12. Nature 307:199 (Jan. 19, 1984)
13. Virkkunen, B.; J. Amer. Med. Assoc. 253(5) 635 (Feb. 1, 1985)
14. Science 227:40–41 (Jan. 4, 1985)
15. Science 227:40–41 (Jan. 4, 1985)
16. Lancet I, 317–318 (1984)
17. Nutr. Week (Sep. 7, 1989)
18. Nutr. Week (September 28, 1989)
19. Nutr. Week (September 21, 1989)
20. Nutr. Week (Nov. 9, 1989)
21. Nutr. Week v17, n30 (1989)

CHAPTER 17

1. Oh, Suk, Y. and Miller, Lorraine T.; Amer. J. Clin. Nutr. 42(3):421–31 (Sep. 1985)
2. Flaim, Evelyn, et al.; Amer. J. Clin. Nutr. 34:1103–8 (June 1981)
3. Nutr. Rev. 43(9) 263–65 (Sep. 1985)
4. Keys, A., et al.; Metabolism 14:759–65 (1965)
5. Kannell, William B. and Gordon, Tavia; USDHEW Report 24 (1970)
6. Nichols, A. B., et al.; Amer. J. Clin. Nutr. 29:1384–92 (1976)
7. Shekelle, R. B., et al.; New Engl. J. Med. 304:65–70 (1981)
8. Drawber, Thomas R., et al.; Amer. J. Clin. Nutr. 36:617–25 (Oct. 1982)
9. Porter, M. W., et al., Amer. J. Clin. Nutr. 30:490–5 (1977)
10. Slater, G., et al.; Nutr. Rep. Internat. 14:249–52 (1976)
11. Kummerow, Fred A., et al.; Amer. J. Clin. Nutr. 30:664–73 (1977)
12. Flynn, M. A., et al.; Amer. J. Clin. Nutr. 32:1051–7 (1979)
13. Hirshowitz, B., et al.; Brit. J. Plastic Surg. 23:529 (1976)
14. Castelli, W. P., et al.; J. Amer. Med. Assoc. 256:2835–8 (Nov. 28, 1986)
15. Naito, J.; Comprehensive Therapy 13(11) 43–52 (Nov. 1987)
16. Press, R. I., Geller, J. and Evans, Gary; Western J. Med. 152:41–45 (1990)

17. Nutr. Today 4 (Sep./Oct. 1989)
18. Nutr. Rep. Intern. 36:641–9 (1987)
19. Brook, J., et al.; Biochem. Med. M. 35:31–9 (1986)
20. Tishikawa et al.; Atherosclerosis 75(2,3):95–104 (Feb. 1989)
21. Sugano, M., et al.; Ann. Nutr. M. 30:289–299 (1986)
22. Hermann, W.; Ann. NY Acad. Sci. 462 (1982)
23. Cloarec, M. J., et al.; Israel J. Med. Sci. 23(8) 869–72 (Aug. 1987)
24. Muckle, Thomas J. and Nazir, Darius J.; Amer. J. Clin. Pathol. 91:165–71 (1989)
25. Ann. Nutr. Metab. 30:94–103 (1986)
26. Gey, F.; Amer. J. Clin. Nutr. 45: 1368–77 (1987)
27. Dallal, G. E., et al.; J. Amer. Coll. Nutr. 8(1)69–74 (Jan. 1989)
28. Chen, L. and Thayer, R.; Nutr. Res. 5:527 (1985)
29. Bazzarre, T.; Nutr. Rep. Int. 33:711–20 (1986)
30. Verlangieri, Anthony J.; FASEB J. 46(5) 595 (1987)
31. DeGroot, A. P. (1963)
32. Luyken, Robert (1965)
33. Kirby, Robert; Amer. J. Clin. Nutr. (1981)
34. Judd, Patricia A.; Amer. J. Clin. Nutr. (1981)
35. Anderson, James; Amer. J. Clin. Nutr. (1984)
36. VanHorn, Linda V.; J. Amer. Dietetic Assoc. (1986)
37. Anderson, James; Amer. Assoc. Cereal Chemists (1986)
38. Turnbull, William; J. Clin. Nutr. & Gastroenterology (1987)
39. VanHorn, Linda V.; J. Prev. Med. (1988)
40. Gold, K. V.; Western J. Med. (1988)
41. Swain, Janis F., et al., New Engl. J. Med. 322(3):147–52 (Jan. 18, 1990)
42. Preventive Medicine (May 1988)
43. Arch. Inter. Med. (Feb. 1988)
44. Pollack, O. J.; Circulation 7:702 (1953)
45. Beveridge, J., Haust, M. & Connell, W.; J. Nutr. 83:119–122 (1964)
46. Matson, F., Grundy, S. and Crouse, J.; Amer. J. Clin. Nutr. 35:697–700 (1982)
47. Nutr. Rev. 45(6) 174–5 (June 1987)
48. Ernst, E.; Pharmathera 5:83–9 (1987)
49. Vacha, G. et al.; Amer. J. Clin. Nutr. 38:532–40 (1983)

50. Prog. Clin. Biol. Res. 125:103–15 (1983)
51. Chem. & Eng. News p69 (Apr. 26, 1986)

CHAPTER 18

1. Panganamala, Rao V. and Cornwell, David G.; in *Vitamin E: Biochemical, Hematological, and Clinical Aspects,* Lubin, Bertram and Machlin, Lawrence J., Eds. Ann. NY Acad. Sci., Vol. 393 (1982)
2. Steiner, Manfred; Thromb. Haemostas 49:73–77 (1983)
3. Reduction of Platelet Adhesiveness by Vitamin E Supplementation in Humans
    Jandak, J., Steiner, Manfred and Richardson, P. D.
    Thrombosis Res. 49:393–404 (1988)
4. Kuo, P., Wilson, A. and Goldstein, R.; J. Amer. Col. Nutr. 3:244 (1984)
5. Srivastava, K.; Pros. Leuk. Med. 21:177–85 (1986)
6. Steiner, Manfred; Tocopherol, Oxygen and Biomembranes, pp 143–63 (1987)
7. Jandak, J., Steiner, Manfred and Richardson, P. D.; Blood 73:141–9 (1989)
8. Norden, R.; Int. J. Micro. 3:425 (1984)
9. Bordia, A. and Verma, S. K.; Clin. Card 8(10) 552–4 (Oct. 1985)
10. Ernst, E.; Pharmathera. 5:83–9 (1987)
11. Bosch, V., et al.; Thromb. Haem 58:165 (1987)
12. Schaefer, A. and Adelman, B.; J. Clin. Invest. 75:456–7 (1985)
13. Taussig, S. and Nieper, H.; J. Int. Assoc. Prev. Med. 6:139–151 (1979)
14. Miyagi, H. et al.; Circulation 79:597–602 (1989)
15. Kok, F. J., et al.; J. Amer. Med. Assoc. 261:1161–4 (1989)
16. Kok, F. J., et al., Amer. J. Clin. Nutr. 45:462–8 (1987)
17. Salonen, J., et al., Atherosclerosis 70:155–60 (1988)
18. Oster, O., et al.; Ann. Clin. Rev. 18:36–42 (1986) [also see Oster, O. and Prellwitz, T.; Biol. Tr. Elem. Res. 24:91–103 (1990)]

CHAPTER 19

1. Bliznakov, Emile and Hunt, Gerald; *The Miracle Nutrient: Coenzyme Q-10* Bantam, NY (1987)
2. Science 211:727–9 (Feb. 13, 1981)
3. Harmesen, E. et al.; Amer. J. Physiol. 246(1 pt 2), H37-H43 (1984)
4. Aviado, A.; J. Pharmacol. 33:546 (1986)
5. Altura, B.; Arch. Inter. Med. (April 1987) [Also see J. Amer. Coll. Nutr. 7:40 (1988)]
6. Altura, Bella and Altura, Burton; Proceed. Nat. Acad. Sci. 87(5) (March 1990)
7. Sjorgren, A., et al.; J. Int. Med. 226:213–222 (1989)
8. Peticone, F., et al.; J. Amer. Coll. Nutr. 7:403 (1988)
9. Curr. Ther. Res. 34:543 (1983)
10. Amer. Heart J. 112:1278 (1986)
11. Dzhaparidze, L. M., et al.; Vopr. Pitan (USSR) 3:41–6 (1986)
12. Frol'kis, V. V., et al.; Fizol. Zh. (Kiev, USSR) 32:24–32 (1986)
13. McLennan, P., et al.; Amer. Heart J. 116:709–717 (1988)

CHAPTER 20

1. Morrison, L.; *Dr. Morrison's Heart-Saver Program*, St. Martin's Press, NY (1982)
2. Morrison, L. M. and Schjeide, O. A.; *Arteriosclerosis: Prevention, treatment, and regression*, Charles A. Thomas, Springfield (1984)
3. Morrison, L. M., Schjeide, O. A. and Meyer, K.; *Coronary Heart Disease and the Mucopolysaccharides*, Charles A. Thomas, Springfield (1974)
4. Nakazawa, K. and Murata, K.; J. Int. Med. Res. 6:217–225 (1978)
5. Miller, N. E. and Lewis, B.; *Lipoprotein, Atherosclerosis and Coronary Heart Disease*, Elsevier/North-Holland Biomedical Press, NY (1981)
6. Horowitz, M. I. and Pigman, W.; *The Glycoconjugates. Vol 2.*, Academic Press, NY (1978)
7. Robinson, R. W.; *Glycosaminoglycans and Arterial Disease*, S. Karger, NY (1975)
8. Varma, R. S. and Varma, R.; *Glycosaminoglycans and*

Proteoglycans in Physiological and Pathological Processes of Body Systems, S. Karger, NY (1982)
9. New England J. Med., 309:396–403 (1983)
10. New Engl. J. Med., pp 262–4 (Jan 28, 1988)

CHAPTER 21

1. Miller, J. Z., et al.; Amer. Heart Assoc. Mtg. (Nov. 1986) [Also see Science News 349 (Nov. 29, 1986)]
2. Matthew 5:13
3. McCarron, D. A., et al.; Sci. 224:1392–8 (June 28, 1984)
4. Priddle, W. (1931), McQuarrie, S., et al. (1936), and Gordon, D. and Drury, D. (1959)
5. Khaw, Kay-Tee, et al.; New Engl. J. Med. 316(5) 235–40 (Jan. 29, 1987)
6. Ueshima, H., et al.; Lancet 1:504 (1981)
7. Beard, T., et al.; Lancet 11:455–8 (1982)
8. MacGregor, G., et al.; Lancet 11:567–70 (1982)
9. Tobian, L., et al.; Hypertension 7(Suppl 1) 1–110—1–114 (1985)
10. Moore, Richard D. and Webb, George D.; *The "K" Factor,* MacMillan, NY (1986) and Pocket Books, NY (1987)
11. McCarron, D. A.; Nutr. Rev. 42:223–25 (June 1984)
12. Parrott-Garcia, M. and McCarron, D. A.; Nutr. Rev. 42:205–13 (June 1984) [Also see Hypertension 7:607–27 (1985)]
13. Johnson, N. E. et al.; Amer. J. Clin. Nutr. 42:12–17 (July 1985)
14. Castenmiller, J. J. M., et al.; Amer. J. Clin. Nutr. 41:52–60 (Jan. 1985)
15. Castenmiller, J. J. M., et al.; J. Epidem. 123(6) (1986)
16. Castenmiller, J. J. M., et al.; Lancet (Sep. 27, 1986)
17. Zemel, M., et al.; Clin. Res. 34:919A (1986)
18. Altura, B. M.; Fed. Proc. 40:2672 (1981)
19. Joffres, Michael R., et al.; Amer. J. Clin. Nutr. 45:469–475 (Feb. 1987)
20. Marier, J. R.; Magnesium 5:1–8 (1986)
21. Larsen, N., et al. (1972)
22. JFASEB (1989)
23. J. Pharm. Exptl. Thera. (1974)
24. Bliznakov, E. and Hunt, G.; *The Miracle Nutrient Co-enzyme Q-10,* pp 110–23, Bantam, NY (1987)

25. Yamagami, T., et al.; *Biomedical and Clinical Aspects of Coenzyme Q*, Vol. 4, pp. 253–262, Elsevier, B. V. (1984)
26. Yamori, Y.; Prog. Clin. Biol. Res. 125:103–15 (1983)
27. Singer, P., et al.; Atherosclerosis 56:111–8 (July 1985)
28. Ibid., 56:223–35 (Aug. 1985)
29. Norris, P. G., et al.; Brit. Med. J. 293:104–5 (July 12, 1986)
30. Knapp, H. and Fitzgerald, G.; New Eng. J. Med. 320(16) 1037–1043 (1989)
31. Ernst, E.; Pharmathera. 5:83–9 (1987)

CHAPTER 22

1. Panush, Richard S.; The Nutrition Report 6(3) 17–20 (1988)
2. Rheumatology News, pp1,4 (July–August, 1982)
3. Sperling, R. I., et al.; Arthritis and Rheumatism 25:133 (1983)
4. Lee, T. H., et al.; New Eng. J. Med. 312(19) 1217–24 (May 9, 1985)
5. Kremer, J., et al.; Clin. Res. 33:A778 (1985)
6. Cleland, L., et al.; J. Rheumatology 15:1471–5 (Oct. 1988)
7. McCormick, J. N., et al.; Lancet 2:508 (1977)
8. Belch, J., et al.; Ann. Rheum. Digest 47:96–104 (1988)
9. Aaseth, J., et al.; *Selenium In Biology and Medicine* (May, 1980)
10. Tarp, U., et al.; Scandinavian J. Rheumatology 14:97–101 (1985)
11. Aaseth, J., et al.; Scandinavian J. Rheumatology 7:237–40 (1978)
12. Mottonen, T., et al.; Clin. Rheumatol. 3:195–200 (1984)
13. Thorling, E. B., et al.; Biol. Tr. Elem. Res. 8:65–73 (1985)
14. Borglund, A., et al.; Scand. J. Clin. Lab. Invest. 48:27–32 (1988)
15. Tarp, U., et al.; Scandinavian J. Rheumatology 14:364–8 (1985)
16. Nutr. Rev. 46(8)284–6 (Aug. 1988)
17. Biol. Tr. Elem. Res. 7:195–198 (May–June 1985)
18. Longevity, p81 (Sep. 1989)
19. Walker, R.; Agents and Actions 76(6);454 (1978)

20.   Charnot, A., et al.; Ann. Endocrinol. 32:397 (1971)
21.   Fredericks, Carlton; *Arthritis: Don't Learn to Live With It,* Grosset & Dunlap, NY (1981)
22.   Lawson, J. W., et al.; 1988 Ann. Mtg. Amer. Soc. Microbiol.

CHAPTER 23

1.   Lafferty, K.; Med. World News (Aug. 25, 1986)
2.   Offenbacher, E.; Diabetes 29:919–25 (1980)
3.   Levine, R. A., et al.; Metabolism 17(2):114–25 (1968)
4.   Doisy, R., *Cowdry's Problems of Aging,* Lansing, ed. Baltimore, Williams Wilkens (1952)
5.   Canfield, W. K. and Doisy, R. J.; Diabetes 24(2):406 (1975)
6.   Evans, G. W.; Int. J. Biosoc. Res. 11(2) 163–180 (1989)
7.   Colette, C., et al., Amer. J. Clin. Nutr. 47:256–261 (Feb. 1988)
8.   Gisinger, C., et al.; Diabetes 37:1260–4 (1988)
9.   Chen, I. and Thacker, R.; Nutr. Res. 5:527–34 (1985)
10.   Dall'Aglio, E., et al.; Int. J. Clin. Pharm., Thera. & Toxicol. 20(3):147–50 (1982)
11.   Steenrod, W. J.; Prevent. Med. 9:423–9 (1966)
12.   Passariello, N., et al.; Internat. J. Clin. Pharm. Therapy & Tox. 21(5) 252–6 (1983)
13.   Passariello, N., et al. (1983)
14.   Hii, C. S. T. and Howell, S. L.; J. Endocr. 107:1–8 (1985)
15.   Cogan, D. G., et al.; Ann. Int. Med. 101:82–91 (1984)
16.   Chaundry, P. S., et al.; Biochem. Pharmacol. 32:1995–8 (1983)
17.   Netherlands J. Med. 29(2) (1986)
18.   Albrink, M. J., et al.; Ann. Mtg. Amer. Diabetes Assoc., Anaheim (1986)
19.   Beard, E. I., et al.; 73rd Ann. FASEB, New Orleans (March 19, 1989)
20.   Mori, T. A. et al., Metabolism 38(5) 404–9 (May 1989)
21.   Esnick, J.; Ann. Mtg. Amer. Diabetes Assoc. (1987)
22.   Glauber, H.; Ann. Mtg. Amer. Diabetes Assoc. (1987)
23.   Pai, Lee H. and Prasad, Ananda S.; Nutr. Res. 8:889–97 (1988)

CHAPTER 24

1. Stewart, A.; J. Reprod. Med. 32(6) 435–41 (1987)
2. Sherwood, R., et al.; Ann. Clin. Bi. 23:667–70 (1986).
3. Abraham, Guy E.; J. Reprod. Med. 28:446–64 (July 1983)
4. London, R. S., et al.; J. Amer. Coll. Nutr. 2:115–22 (April–June 1983)
5. London, R. S., et al.; J. Reprod. Med. 32:400–4 (1987)
6. Vorherr, Helmuth; VERIS Vitamin E Seminar (April 30, 1986)
7. Kendall, Kim E. and Schnurr, Paula P.; Obstetrics and Gynecology 70:145–9 (Aug. 1987)
8. Brush, M. and Perry, M.; Lancet I:1399 (1985)
9. Brush, M., et al.; Brit. J. Clin. Path. 42:448–52 (1988)
10. Williams, M., et al.; J. Int. Med. R. 13:174–9 (1985)
11. Horrobin, David; J. Reprod. Med. 28:6,465–468 (1983)
12. Brush, M.; Amer. J. Obst. Gyn. 150:363–366 (1984)
13. Dupont, W. D. and Page, D. L.; New Engl. J. Med. 312:146–51 (Jan. 17, 1985)
14. Parrazinni, F., et al.; Surgery 99:576 (1986)
15. London, R. S., et al.; Nutr. Res. 2:243–7 (1982)
16. London, R. S., et al.; Obstet. Gynecol. 59:519–23 (1981)
17. Abrams, A. A.; New Engl. J. Med. 272:1080–1

CHAPTER 25

1. Pauling, Linus; *How to Live Longer and Feel Better,* Freeman and Co., New York (1986)
2. Lee, Janda; Center for Health Science News, Univ. Wisconsin at Madison, 2–4 (Nov. 12, 1987)
3. Johnston, C.; J. Amer. Coll. Nutr. 9:150–9 (1990)

CHAPTER 27

1. *Recommended Dietary Allowances,* Subcommittee on the Tenth Edition of the RDAs, Food and Nutrition Board, Commission on Life Sciences, National Research Council, National Academy Press, Wash. D. C. (1989)

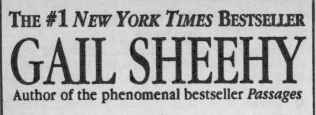

THE
SUPERMARKET
NUTRITION
COUNTER

Annette Natow, Ph.D.,R.D.,
and Jo-Ann Heslin, M.A.,R.D.

Bestselling Authors of
The Fat Counter* and *The Cholesterol Counter

POCKET
BOOKS

Barnes & Noble, Inc.
Metro Center
10235 N. Metro Pkwy East
Phoenix, AZ 85051
602-678-0088 03-08-00 S02560 R006

CUSTOMER RECEIPT COPY

New Super-Nutrition   6.99
0671700715

SUBTOTAL   6.99
SALES TAX   .50
TOTAL   7.49
AMOUNT TENDERED
MASTERCARD   7.49
CARD #:   5300000891364115
EXP DATE   0602
AMOUNT   7.49
AUTH CODE   089440

TOTAL PAYMENT   7.49
Thanks for shopping at Barnes & Noble!
#23364 03-08-00 04:02P Dana

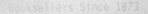

Booksellers Since 1873

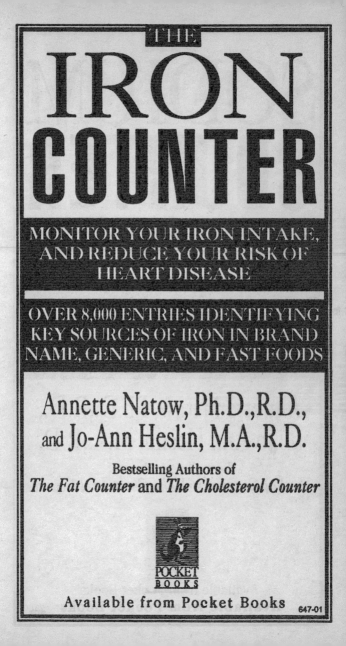

THE
IRON
COUNTER

MONITOR YOUR IRON INTAKE, AND REDUCE YOUR RISK OF HEART DISEASE

OVER 8,000 ENTRIES IDENTIFYING KEY SOURCES OF IRON IN BRAND NAME, GENERIC, AND FAST FOODS

Annette Natow, Ph.D.,R.D., and Jo-Ann Heslin, M.A.,R.D.

Bestselling Authors of
The Fat Counter and *The Cholesterol Counter*

POCKET
BOOKS

Available from Pocket Books   647-01

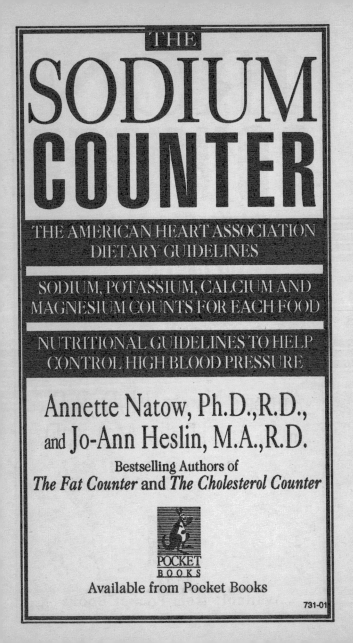

THE
SODIUM
COUNTER

THE AMERICAN HEART ASSOCIATION DIETARY GUIDELINES

SODIUM, POTASSIUM, CALCIUM AND MAGNESIUM COUNTS FOR EACH FOOD

NUTRITIONAL GUIDELINES TO HELP CONTROL HIGH BLOOD PRESSURE

Annette Natow, Ph.D.,R.D., and Jo-Ann Heslin, M.A.,R.D.

Bestselling Authors of
The Fat Counter and *The Cholesterol Counter*

POCKET
BOOKS

Available from Pocket Books

731-01